Understanding Aging, Fatigue, and Inflammation

Rainer H. Straub

Understanding Aging, Fatigue, and Inflammation

When the Immune System and Brain Compete for Energy in the Body

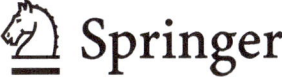

Rainer H. Straub
Department of Internal Medicine
University Hospital Regensburg
Regensburg, Germany

ISBN 978-3-662-68903-5   ISBN 978-3-662-68904-2   (eBook)
https://doi.org/10.1007/978-3-662-68904-2

Translation from the German language edition: "Altern, Müdigkeit und Entzündungen verstehen" by Rainer H. Straub, © Springer-Verlag GmbH Deutschland 2018. Published by Springer Berlin Heidelberg. All Rights Reserved.

This book is a translation of the original German edition "Altern, Müdigkeit und Entzündungen verstehen" by Rainer H. Straub, published by Springer-Verlag GmbH, DE in 2018. The translation was done with the help of an artificial intelligence machine translation tool. A subsequent human revision was done primarily in terms of content, so that the book will read stylistically differently from a conventional translation. Springer Nature works continuously to further the development of tools for the production of books and on the related technologies to support the authors.

Photo credits cover: Reicher/Stock.adobe.com
This Springer imprint is published by the registered company Springer-Verlag GmbH, DE, part of Springer Nature.
The registered company address is: Heidelberger Platz 3, 14197 Berlin, Germany

Paper in this product is recyclable.

The misfortune of the creature is the unwanted energy expenditure that prevents desired energy expenditures for physical and mental efforts.

For Jürgen Schölmerich,
a friend and supporter of lateral thinking

Foreword

The digitized world brings with it the fact that via Facebook, WhatsApp, blog pages, and many other variants, writing activity on even the most irrational topics is constantly increasing and is omnipresent. A significant disadvantage of this is that while an unmanageable amount of short communication messages and comments flow through the air or the earth cables, a meaningful context to overarching topics is rarely discernible. Sustainability is also usually not recognizable in this, although there might possibly be some clever ideas behind it if one were to think them through to the end and also put them into words.

Exactly this path has been taken by one of the most innovative minds of our time, my long-time colleague and friend, Rainer H. Straub—once again—by summarizing and channeling ubiquitous questions and unsolved mysteries, thus opening a new perspective for the inclined readers.

In this book, the brain and immune system compete, allowing us to sense how much contradiction operates within our body and how much these two "egoists" depend on each other. This problem can be understood especially in conversations with patients with systemic-inflammatory immunological diseases every day, as hardly any of these patients report that they are fully mentally and physically capable despite their disease being inactive under therapy, even though "all" (laboratory) parameters show no activity of their inflammatory disease. This reflects the "concept of the two realms" also contemplated and newly formulated by the author, guided by egotists (brain and immune system) who assist each other in energetic emergencies, but still compete for the limited resources in the body in the long term.

The imbalance of the energy balance and the resulting problems are therefore also the central intersection of this book, and it is very interesting to trace how the author transforms this wealth of information into sometimes deliberately humorous, but easily understandable streams of thought and reading.

For those who are not only interested in the basic culture of conflict between the two egoists (brain and immune system), but also in practical examples and many explanations of individual symptoms and disease states, the third part of the book is intended, in which the individual problems of this energetic imbalance are explained in detail. A special feature is that the author, although he is not yet to be classified in this age group, provides an outlook on the egoistic-energetic processes with increasing age and explains comprehensibly why due to these processes physical youthfulness cannot always be maintained. However, since this only applies to a limited extent to the brain, every interested person is advised to read this work. The mental performance of the reader, even in old age, will certainly be sustainably supported by reading this book.

With special thanks to Rainer H. Straub and his not insignificant efforts to write this work.

Ulf Müller-Ladner
Bad Nauheim/Gießen
im Herbst 2017

Preface

With the description of the genetic material (DNA) in the 1950s, we experienced an unprecedented **molecular revolution**. True to the motto "Everything is molecule and molecule is everything", many scientists lose themselves in details. Since then, biomedical science has increasingly focused on tiny individual parts of the cell machinery, and the view of the whole is often lost. The patient laments this.

Clinically active, researching physicians, who actually always consider the entire human being and not just a single cell, adhere to this **detail-oriented thinking**. Therefore, research projects often have a single molecule at their center. Even epidemiologically oriented physicians (human geneticists) focus on a tiny genetic detail in order to relate it to diseases in population-based studies using mathematical methods. This focus on detail leads to the problem of a clear description of the transition from cellular events to the problem for the entire human being, the symptom. The patient experiences or feels a symptom, and from there it is a long way to the interior of a cell and to the molecule.

Thus, there are **symptoms** such as depressive mood, fatigue, sleep disorders, loss of appetite and the associated malnutrition and undernutrition, muscle atrophy, bone loss, weight gain and weight loss, dwindling libido and reduced fertility, high blood pressure, increased blood clotting, back pain and much more. Of course, cellular and molecular processes are behind this, but describing the transitions from the intracellular to the whole is extremely difficult. This is probably because we have so far hardly developed a scientific method for assessing and describing the whole. However, in the last two decades, physicians, psychologists, and natural scientists have made important progress by relating various research areas to each other (this began in Germany in the early 1990s).

On the one hand, this is the field of **Psycho-Neuro-Endocrino-Immunology**, where the linking factors between the brain and body—namely nerve fibers (Neuro), hormonal glands (Endocrino) and immune cells (Immuno)—are considered. In doing so, these researchers draw on molecular insights from the individual sub-disciplines, focus on the linking paths between the organ systems, and thus consider the whole. In the USA, this field is often referred to as Mind-Body Medicine today.

Furthermore, in the last two decades, the field of **Evolutionary Medicine** has emerged, adopting the concepts of evolutionary biology for medicine. Evolutionary medicine provides an extraordinarily valuable perspective on the whole. It explains relationships by asserting that they must have a benefit in the context of reproduction (English: "fitness"). If a benefit arises for the individual, genes and the pathways dependent on them are conserved in the gene pool of the offspring. Over many generations, this phylogenetic development leads to traits that exist today (including genes and molecules in us humans), which have a measurable benefit in the context of reproduction. The individual molecule, the gene, or entire signaling pathways, which we usually consider in the context of a disease, probably have entirely different roles in the context of reproduction, for which they were positively selected. Evolutionary medicine sharpens this view, thus creating a new approach to the whole.

Then there is the field of **energy regulation**, which deals more closely with the body's energy supply. Hardly any process in our body takes place without energy, which is why energy-rich substrates must be constantly supplied. However, energy is also constantly lost for heat production and many other functions. Energy-rich substrates are glucose, fatty acids, and proteins, from which cellular energy is obtained. Thus, energy intake and energy expenditure take place at the level of a single cell, but also at the level of the entire body. The energy consumption and energy intake of the human body can be determined exactly using scientifically flawless methods, so that we get a wonderful view of the whole with these procedures.

Within psycho-neuro-endocrino-immunology, many pathways can be explained by the fact that they serve the **energy regulation of the entire body** and reproduction. Starting from the physical role of energy, the first part of the book deals with energy regulation of the entire body. Furthermore, evolutionary medicine is presented, which provides valuable insights throughout the book. The second part of the book presents energy expenditures for various aspects such as immune defense, pain, psychological stress, sleep disorders, anxiety, and others in more detail. With this information, a connection between energy regulation, evolutionary medicine, and the above-mentioned symptoms is made in the third part of the book. The fourth part summarizes everything. Following the text, there is an appendix with a glossary that explains important terms in detail. In addition, there is an extensive keyword index attached.

The author worked for many years in the field of Psycho-Neuro-Endocrino-Immunology (specifically in relation to chronic inflammatory diseases), to then integrate the two elements of evolutionary medicine and energy regulation. This book was created with the desire to represent a transition between molecular and holistic medicine. The content should remain as simple as possible. This may not always have been successful, although a lot of help flowed in from outside.

Such a book is never created entirely on its own, and therefore here too a few very helpful people have given good advice for the German version of the book. The book was critically read and significantly improved, making it more generally understandable. We scientists live in an ivory tower, and we are so blinkered that we urgently need this help. In this sense, the book was read by Dr. Anne Asmacher, Dr. Hubert Stangl, Verena Straub and Gabriele Konanz. Valuable help also came from the Springer publishing house from Dr. Christine Lerche and Claudia Bauer. If inclined readers provide further tips, the author is grateful, because improvements are collected and then added in a further edition.

Rainer H.Straub
Regensburg
im Herbst 2017

Contents

I   Energy, Evolution and Medicine

1   **Energy and Body** 3
1.1   The Pfühlbach and the Dispute... 5
1.2   Of Reservoirs and Bicycle Dynamos... 6
1.3   Stories of Thermos Flasks... 7
1.4   What is Vital Force?.. 7
1.5   The Human Body—An Open System 9
1.6   CAEN ("Controllable Amount of Energy") or How Much Energy Does the
       Body Need? 12
1.7   The Big Three 15
1.8   Why We Store Energy—Fever, Tour de France and Newborns 15
1.9   How Much Energy Do We and Our Ancestor Australopithecus Store?................ 18
1.10   Sweet Tooth—Brain, Muscles, and Immune System 21
1.11   Food Search Prior to Energy Storage 22
1.12   Neuronal Factors and Hormones of Energy Storage 23
1.13   A Little Lesson on Stress Hormones 26
1.14   A Brief Lesson on Immune Messengers.. 27
1.15   Stress Hormones and Cytokines Release Energy................................. 27
1.16   A New Look at the CAEN ("Controllable Amount of Energy")...................... 31
       References 33

2   **Evolutionary Medicine**.. 35
2.1   Darwin, Wallace & Co.—Simultaneity of a Discovery............................ 36
2.2   Darwinian Evolution—Species and Selection................................... 37
2.3   Darwinian Evolution—Modern Additions 38
2.4   Chickens from Behind... 39
2.5   Founder Effect in Canada, Lactose Intolerance and Fat Babies................. 42
2.6   The Selfish Brain.. 44
2.7   The Selfish Immune System 46
2.8   When Two Fight 47
       References 49

3   **Brain and Immune System—Two Competing Realms**.................................. 51
3.1   Energy Release—Competing Role of Brain and Immune System.................... 52
3.2   Energy Release—Mutual Immediate Assistance 54
3.3   Energy Storage—Memory Function of Brain and Immune System.................. 55
       References 60

II   Energy Expenditure in the Spotlight

4   **Inflammation and Energy** 63
4.1   Historical Definition of Inflammation 64
4.2   Inflammation Strength: Rose Thorn, Rheumatism, and Sepsis 65

4.3	Inflammation Causes Increased Energy Expenditure	67
	References	72

5	**Pain and Energy**	73
5.1	The Pain Receptors and Pain Stabilization	74
5.2	Inflammation Causes Pain—The Sixth Sense	75
5.3	When the Muscle Becomes Acidic, It Hurts	76
5.4	Heat, Cold, and Pepper—Where Does It Reach the Brain?	76
5.5	Acute and Chronic Pain	77
5.6	Electric Shock, Pain, and Energy Expenditure	78
5.7	Heat, Cold and Energy Expenditure	79
	References	80

6	**Psychological Stress and Energy**	83
6.1	What is Stress?	84
6.2	Acute Stress—Sport as a Model	84
6.3	Chronic Stress is Unhealthy	85
6.4	Chronic Stress at Work	86
6.5	Stressful Double Hits	87
6.6	Psychological Stress Causes Increased Energy Expenditure	87
6.7	Dementia and Heart Disease Increase Energy Expenditure	88
	References	89

7	**Other Energy-Consuming Situations**	91
7.1	Sleep Problems—Sleep Apnea	92
7.2	Chronic Smoldering Infections	92
7.3	Fear and Anxiety	94
7.4	6 Cigarettes per Day	95
	References	96

8	**What Does Increased Energy Expenditure Mean for the Body?**	99
8.1	Energy Expenditure in Aging	101
8.2	Energy Expenditure is Hereditary	103
8.3	Energy Situation During Aging with Additional Energy Expenditures	104
	References	107

III   From Energy and Evolution to Symptom

9	**Daytime Fatigue and Depression**	111
9.1	Sickness Behavior in Chronic Inflammatory Disease	112
9.2	Daytime Fatigue and Depression in Old Age	114
	References	115

10	**Sleep Disorders and Circadian Symptoms**	117
10.1	How can Sleep be Studied?	118
10.2	Sleep and Circadian Rhythms in Chronic Inflammatory Diseases	119
10.3	Circadian Rhythm of Inflammation	120
10.4	Sleep Problems in Old Age	123
	References	124

11	**Loss of Appetite, Malnutrition, and Undernutrition**	125
11.1	Appetite and Chronic Inflammation	126
11.2	Anorexia of Aging	127
	References	128
12	**Muscle Loss**	129
12.1	Muscle Loss and Chronic Inflammation	130
12.2	Detour: Nutrition and Chronic Inflammation	132
12.3	Muscle Mass Decreases with Age	132
	References	135
13	**Bone Loss—Osteoporosis**	137
13.1	Bone Loss and Chronic Inflammation	138
13.2	Bone Loss in Old Age	140
	References	141
14	**Weight Changes (Increase and Decrease)**	143
14.1	Weight and Chronic Inflammation	144
14.2	Weight During Aging	144
	References	154
15	**The Storage Hormone Insulin Doesn't Work—Insulin Resistance**	157
15.1	Antonin Sulin in Resistance	158
15.2	Storage in Chronic Inflammation—Role of Insulin	158
15.3	Insulin Resistance in Aging	159
	References	161
16	**Decreasing Libido, Lower Fertility**	163
16.1	Sex and Chronic Inflammation	164
16.2	Of Antechinus, Sea Elephants, and Macaques	165
16.3	Estrogens and Chronic Inflammation	166
16.4	Hormones in Old Age	167
	References	168
17	**Sympathetic Nervous System Fires and Causes High Blood Pressure**	169
17.1	Cortisol and Inflammation	170
17.2	Cooperation of Stress Hormones and Consequence in Chronic Inflammation	171
17.3	Sympathetic Nervous System and Aging	173
17.4	Low Activity of the Parasympathetic Nervous System	173
	References	175
18	**Increased Blood Clotting—Thrombosis/Embolism**	177
18.1	Coagulation Explained: Lampreys, Sea Squirts, Fugu, and Humans	178
18.2	Coagulation and Inflammation	180
18.3	Increased Coagulation in Chronic Inflammation	181
18.4	Acceleration of Coagulation in Old Age	182
	References	182
19	**Stress Worsens Inflammation, and Inflammation Alters Stress Tolerance**	185
19.1	Stress and Factor X Constitute a Double Hit	186
19.2	Anti-Stress Therapies	187

19.3   Stress in the Elderly 188
        References 190

IV   The Big Summary

20   **The Synthesis** 195
20.1   Addition of Energy Forms and Unwanted Energy Expenditure...................... 196
20.2   What are Telomeres? 198
20.3   Inflammation, Cell Turnover and Telomere Length 199
20.4   Chronic Inflammation and Telomere Length 199
20.5   Pain, Stress and Telomere Length 200
20.6   Anxiety, Smoking, and Telomere Length 201
20.7   Conclusion 202
        References 202

        Supplementary Information
        Appendix 206

List of Figures

Fig. 1.1   Examples of forms of energy in an isolated system   8
Fig. 1.2   Structure of a dextrose molecule (called glucose)   10
Fig. 1.3   Breakdown of the main energy-rich substrates in food within a cell   11
Fig. 1.4   Comparison of energy expenditures per day in healthy humans at
various activities (4,1868 kJ = 1 kcal)   13
Fig. 1.5   Energy stores in the human body.   20
Fig. 1.6   Messenger substances in the human body—short and long-distance
effects   22
Fig. 1.7   Significance of the vagus nerve and insulin for body weight.   23
Fig. 1.8   Regulation of energy storage in the human body   25
Fig. 1.9   Regulation of energy release in the human body.   30
Fig. 2.1   Systematics in the animal kingdom with a special focus on the species
"Homo sapiens"   38
Fig. 2.2   Distribution of milk tolerance around the world   43
Fig. 3.1   The two realms of acute energy provision (upper half) in contrast
to the long-term program of energy storage (lower half)   53
Fig. 3.2   a, b Spatial structure of tetanus toxin (a foreign antigen) and
insulin (b autoantigen)   57
Fig. 4.1   a, b Typical changes in severe joint inflammation named rheumatoid
arthritis. a Joint deformation. b Redness and swelling as well as nodules
along the extensor tendons of muscles that move the fingers (rheumatoid
nodules)   65
Fig. 4.2   Serum levels of Interleukin-6 in different states   67
Fig. 4.3   Increase in Interleukin-6 levels increases energy expenditure per day.   68
Fig. 4.4   Correlation between the blood levels of C-reactive protein and the
energy expenditure per day in patients with rheumatoid arthritis.   71
Fig. 5.1   Pain receptor at the end of a pain nerve fiber   74
Fig. 5.2   Representation of the various body areas in the cerebral cortex   77
Fig. 8.1   Energy expenditure under various conditions   100
Fig. 8.2   Energy expenditure during the aging process. (Data from Speakman
and Westerterp 2010)   102
Fig. 8.3   Energy expenditure during the aging process with simultaneous
additional unwanted energy expenditure.   105
Fig. 9.1   a, b Energy saving through sleep. a Total energy expenditure, b Glucose
consumption by the brain. (Data from Ravussin et al. 1986; Boyle et al.
1994)   113
Fig. 10.1 a–c Circadian rhythm of joint stiffness, pain, and physical dysfunctions
in rheumatoid arthritis. (Data from Straub and Cutolo 2007)   119
Fig. 10.2 Circadian rhythm of Interleukin-6 in patients with rheumatoid arthritis
and healthy normal individuals. (Data from Straub and Cutolo 2007) . . .   121
Fig. 10.3 Circadian rhythm of cortisol and adrenaline/noradrenaline.   122
Fig. 10.4 Increasing sleep problems in old age. (Data from Roberts et al. 2000)   123
Fig. 12.1 Causes of muscle loss.   134
Fig. 13.1 Causes of inflammation-related bone loss.   140

Fig. 14.1   Percentage of people over the age of 15 with obesity.
             (Data from the Organisation for Economic Co-operation
             and Development—OECD 2014)   146
Fig. 14.2   Vicious cycle of weight gain.   152
Fig. 15.1   Factors that can lead to insulin resistance and hyperinsulinemia   161
Fig. 16.1   Influence of the inflammation factor interleukin-6 on the serum
             levels of testosterone. (Data from Tsigos et al. 1999)   164
Fig. 18.1   Blood coagulation in the human body.   179
Fig. 19.1   Significance of Factor X in stress and inflammation.   188
Fig. 19.2   Double hit of mutual reinforcement of inflammation and psychological
             stress   189
Fig. 20.1   Optimal relationship between lifetime and well-being/health   197
Fig. 20.2   Telomere and Telomerase.   198

List of Tables

Table 1.1   Total energy expenditure in various situations and energy
              expenditure of organs and organ systems in a human during a
              day (180 cm and 85 kg)   16
Table 1.2   Energy storage and emaciation time in our ancestors, in modern
              humans, in the domestic pig, and in the chicken   19
Table 1.3   Regulation of energy storage and energy release in the
              human body.   31
Table 2.1   Distance between humans and the last common ancestors of the
              mentioned species in years   41
Table 6.1   What is addition and what is synergism?   87
Table 14.1   Characteristics of chronically stressed individuals who gain or
              lose weight   149
Table 20.1   Unwanted energy expenditures as a percentage of total
              energy expenditure.   201

Energy, Evolution and Medicine

The book aims to provide a comprehensible explanation of typical problems associated with aging and chronic inflammation. These problems were mentioned in the preface, and fatigue is such a critical and central symptom that it made it into the title of the book. However, before we can reach the level of understanding these elements in Parts II and III of the book, we need to acquire the necessary tools in Part I.

▶ Chapter 1 begins with the physical consideration of energy. It describes the energy-rich substrates important to us humans (glucose, fatty acids, and proteins), the energy expenditure of the human body, and the body's own regulation of energy storage and energy release. It becomes clear that the brain and the immune system are the main consumers of energy. The 1st chapter of Part I is challenging, and perhaps one might need to read it twice, but it is the important platform for the rest of the book.

▶ Chapter 2 summarizes—starting from the two discoverers Darwin and Wallace—the contents of the modern theory of evolution and the significance of evolutionary biology for medicine. Evolutionary biological examples are presented that are relevant to today's human medicine. From the special roles of the brain and immune system, the energy egoism of these two organ systems is derived. And it becomes clear that the brain and the immune system dominate the energy regulation.

▶ Chapter 3 demonstrates the special roles of the brain and immune system and explains the memory function of both in the context of the energy question. It presents the competition between the two organ systems, but also the mutual immediate assistance in energy regulation.

Part I summarizes the mechanisms of energy regulation dominated by the brain and immune system.

Energy and Body

Contents

1.1   The Pfühlbach and the Dispute – 5

1.2   Of Reservoirs and Bicycle Dynamos – 6

1.3   Stories of Thermos Flasks – 7

1.4   What is Vital Force? – 7

1.5   The Human Body—An Open System – 9

1.6   CAEN ("Controllable Amount of Energy") or How Much
        Energy Does the Body Need? – 12

1.7   The Big Three – 15

1.8   Why We Store Energy—Fever, Tour de France
        and Newborns – 15

1.9   How Much Energy Do We and Our Ancestor
        Australopithecus Store? – 18

1.10   Sweet Tooth—Brain, Muscles, and Immune System – 21

1.11   Food Search Prior to Energy Storage – 22

1.12   Neuronal Factors and Hormones of Energy Storage – 23

1.13   A Little Lesson on Stress Hormones – 26

1.14   A Brief Lesson on Immune Messengers – 27

1.15   Stress Hormones and Cytokines Release Energy – 27

1.16   A New Look at the CAEN ("Controllable Amount of Energy") – 31

References – 33

1.1 **The Pfühlbach and the Dispute**

The ten-year-old son of a pharmacist, Robert, played at the Pfühlbach, a small river near Heilbronn that flows into the river Neckar. He passionately built simple water mills, dreaming of inventing a *perpetual motion machine*. A perpetual motion machine is a utopian machine that performs work indefinitely without an energy supply. It would have been something if Robert had invented such a machine. He conducted many experiments, only to have to admit with a heavy heart that a *perpetual motion machine* could not be built. These experiments never left Robert. Many mill wheels ran hot and left a lasting memory in him: "Mechanical work and the associated heat cannot be created out of nothing."

The interest of Julius Robert Mayer (1814–1877) did not come out of nowhere, as his father instilled in him a love for science. Mayer Senior filled the house to the brim with various chemical and physical instruments, botanical and mineralogical collections, medicinal plants, and many books. Robert often accompanied his father on excursions, and gradually began to conduct chemical and physical experiments on his own.

Nevertheless, Robert Mayer did not choose a natural science subject, but instead studied medicine, which he completed in March 1839. After a one-year adventure as a ship's doctor aboard the *Java* in the East Indian Ocean, Mayer began to ponder important questions of physics from 1840 onwards. Analogous to the indestructibility of matter, he was fascinated by the topic of the indestructibility of physical forces, and he summarized these considerations in a first publication in June 1841 at the age of 27. Indestructibility meant for him that a force (cause) produces an effect (result), so that this effect generates a new force that produces a next effect, and so on. Everything should be traceable back to a primal force. Energy or work in the modern physical sense was not yet spoken of at that time.

This first attempt at publication in the *Annalen der Physik und Chemie*, the most important German publication organ in the natural sciences of his time, was unsuccessful, as the editor Johann Christian Poggendorf never responded despite receiving three letters from Mayer. The following year, Mayer published the slightly modified text in the *Annalen der Chemie* under the editorship of Justus Liebig. In principle, this early work already discusses energy conservation and energy transfer—for example, from mechanical processes to heat.

Through elegant analogies and thought experiments, Mayer succeeded in establishing a correct relationship between the mechanical work of lifting a weight and the work of heating a quantity of gas. He calculated that a 1 gram body would have to be lifted and dropped 367 meters (mechanical work) to heat one cubic centimeter of air from an initial temperature of 0 degrees Celsius to 1 degree. Work and heat were thus closely related, and he had correctly recognized this. He himself always referred to this relationship as "the mechanical equivalent of heat." One can easily imagine how complicated wooden constructions of mill wheels in the Pfühlbach slowly heated up or even smoked. This must have deeply imprinted itself on him.

Mayer himself never used the terms work or energy, which were only later introduced by other physicists such as Rudolf Clausius, James Joule, William Thomson (Lord Kelvin), William Rankine, and others. Nevertheless, he succeeded in describing the principle of energy conservation and "the mechanical equivalent of heat" for the first time. From 1848, he argued with James Joule for several years over the

1

priority of the first description. Ultimately, this dispute was never sufficiently re-solved, as depending on the scientific camp, either Mayer (the German side) or Joule (the English side) are named as the discoverer of energy conservation.

Hermann von Helmholtz also investigated similar questions within physiology at the end of the 1840s and wrote a paper "On the Conservation of Force," which was equally rejected by Poggendorf. Helmholtz and Mayer also had a dispute over this work due to intellectual property theft. These priority disputes were often also a national issue in the nineteenth century, which was publicly discussed, so that the respective scientist of a nation was often locally highly honored to increase the con-trast to the co-discoverer of another nation. Mayer and von Helmholtz received several German prizes and honorary doctorates during their lifetime. The same was true for James Joule and others in Great Britain. Julius Robert Mayer died of tu-berculosis at the age of 63 (1877). In the end, James Joule won the race because it is called Kilojoule and not Kilomayer.

1.2 Of Reservoirs and Bicycle Dynamos

Energy is a central physical quantity (unit: Joule or Kilojoule). With energy, work can be done, and work is the product of force and distance. For example, a stone that has been rolled up a mountain with a lot of force and over a long distance contains energy:

Force [unit: Newton] × Distance [unit: Meter]

This energy is released again when it rolls down. Or there is "clean" energy in the water of a reservoir, which is led down into the valley via pipes and drives tur-bines and generators.

Energy comes in different forms (see infobox "Explanation").

Explanation: Forms of Energy and Examples
- Potential Energy (the example of the stone on the mountain or water in the reser-voir)
- Kinetic Energy (energy of a moving body)
- Rotational Energy (kinetic energy in a rotating body)
- Elastic Energy (energy in a stretched spring)
- Thermal Energy (kinetic energy of particles in gas, liquid or solids)
- Chemical Energy (energy that is generated in a chemical reaction e.g. heat or movement)
- Electrical Energy (energy that is in electric current and electric fields)
- Magnetic Energy (energy in magnetic fields)
- Electromagnetic Energy (energy in visible and invisible radiation, solar energy)
- Quantum Energy (energy in a light quantum [photon])
- and others

No matter what form of energy is present: The important thing is that work can be done using this energy. Energy can be converted from one form to another. For example, the potential energy of a stone on a mountain can at least partially be transferred into the kinetic energy of the stone as it rolls down. Another part of the energy is converted into heat through friction. Steam engines convert heat into mechanical energy, and bicycle dynamos convert mechanical energy into electrical energy (current flows), which is then converted into heat and electromagnetic energy in the bicycle's light bulb (light is produced). During the conversion, there are always significant losses, so that often heat—as with the light bulb—is given off (another example: When the stone rolls down the mountain, this leads to the generation of frictional heat on the ground and on the stone).

1.3 Stories of Thermos Flasks

If one imagines oneself in a thought experiment in a building similar to a perfect thermos flask, so that exchange with the environment is completely prevented, then neither energy can be given off nor taken up. We call it an isolated system. In reality, such isolated systems do not exist, and therefore we also resorted to the thought experiment. If the thermos flask can hold the heat for hours, tiny particles can still penetrate the wall of the thermos flask, and energy can thus be exchanged with the environment.

But let's continue to assume that we are in such an isolated system (◘ Fig. 1.1), then forms of energy within this system can be converted into each other. But no energy can be lost or newly created, or in other words, it cannot be destroyed or created out of nothing. And to put it another way: "The energy in an isolated system is constant." This is exactly what the law of conservation of energy expresses. Therefore, the production of a utopian machine that performs work permanently without energy input (*perpetual motion machine*) is impossible, because more than the existing energy cannot arise out of nothing from the constant energy in the system. In the ideal thermos flask, it remains at best always the same temperature.

At this point, it is time for us to say goodbye to the isolated system of the thermos flask and the thought experiment and to look at open systems such as a human body. But before that, some basic considerations need to be made.

1.4 What is Vital Force?

Since earliest times, it was assumed that many phenomena of living organisms cannot be described with the laws of inanimate objects. Thus, special causes and forces were assumed in living bodies, which were supposed to be responsible for these phenomena. These were fictitious forces that were not based on chemical-physical laws. The example of sea urchin development, described by the German biologist Hans Driesch (1867–1941), is given.

Hans Driesch began studying at the University of Jena in 1887. He received his doctorate in 1889, and after some travels on the eastern sea, he ended up at the world-famous *Stazione Zoologica* in Naples. There, marine biology was and still is the focus, and so Hans Driesch came to study the development of sea urchins. Sea urchin eggs develop similarly to human embryos, from a two-cell stage to a four-cell stage to an eight-cell stage and so on. At the two-cell stage, Driesch separated the two connected sister cells and observed their further development. He recognized

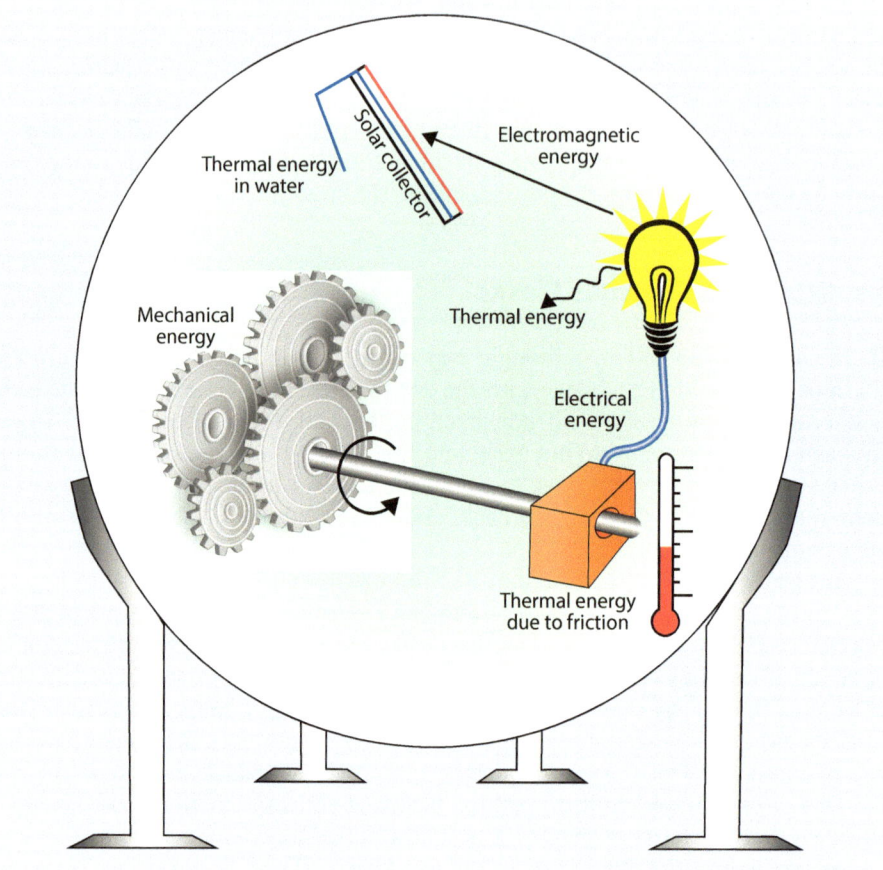

Examples of forms of energy in an isolated system. Forms of energy can be converted into each other, but the total energy of the isolated system remains constant. Nothing is added and nothing is lost.

■ **Fig. 1.1**   Examples of forms of energy in an isolated system

that separated cells developed into a complete sea urchin, as if the cells had never been separated. This was a fascinating circumstance that required an explanation. Stimulated by philosophical considerations, Driesch now assumed that in each part of the sea urchin a real factor—let's call it factor D—would be effective, working on behalf of the whole and controlling the growth process. This factor D must also be active in any substance renewal in the sense of wound healing.

This factor D was named quite differently by other researchers. For example, Hippocrates (ca. 400 BC) called it "physis" (nature), Aristotle (ca. 350 BC) called it "origin, motion and moving", van Helmont (1580–1644) called it "archea", Descartes (1596–1650) spoke of "esprits-animaux", Kaau-Boerhaave (1715–1758) called it "impetum faciens", Bergson (1859–1941) spoke of "élan vital", others referred to it as soul, primum movens, vis essentialis, vis insita, vis vitae, vital principle, vital force, Vitalism, and so on.

Life should have certain inherent laws and thus not be directly accessible to scientific research forever and ever (so the proponents). In Germany, the term vital force gained strong momentum in the era of German Idealism, among other things through Schelling's philosophy of nature (end of the eighteenth century to the first third of the nineteenth century). Even today, this factor D still has significance, especially in Central Europe, much less so in the Anglo-American countries.

This vital force was still a common explanatory principle for many phenomena in medicine and biology in the times of Robert Mayer. Even the great German physiologist Johannes Müller (1801–1858) used terms like vital principle, vis essentialis and others in his *Handbook of Human Physiology*, which was published in the 1830s. Only from the 1840s onwards, the term vital force was increasingly avoided. At the same time, the ideas about different forms of energy within human medicine became more and more prevalent (heat, movement through muscle work, heart work). Here, the "factor D" was then more and more a physical quantity.

Regarding these new thoughts, Robert Mayer, Hermann von Helmholtz and Theodor Schwann were particularly leading within German physiology. They abandoned the obscure concept of force and replaced it with fundamental physical-chemical principles (see infobox "Explanation").

Explanation: Alternative Energy Concepts

At this point, it should be noted that the energy in the human body is a measurable physical quantity, there to perform physical work in some way:

Work = Force × Distance [Unit: Newton × Meter].

In various yoga directions, in Chinese medicine and in alternative medicine, concepts of energy are represented such as "*Kundalini Yoga* to increase the human energy level", "Prana", invisible "energy flows in the body", "holistic energy medicine", "energy centers of the body", "life energy", "energy work and self-resonance", "personal energy management", "Qi" and so on.

For medicine in terms of physical quantities and chemical-physical processes, these terms have no significance. These energy concepts are to be considered in the same sense as the already mentioned vital force. Those who find them a source of orientation and support may use them.

1.5 The Human Body—An Open System

Now we return to the isolated and the open system. The human body is an open system, and it has a lively exchange with the environment, so that energy in the form of heat energy is lost over the surface or chemical energy must be taken in through food. The human body is not a utopian machine (*perpetual motion machine*), for it does not run out of nothing. The body relies on energy supply.

When eating and drinking, we consume three fundamentally different nutrients, namely

- Carbohydrates (building block: e.g. dextrose),
- Fats (building block: fatty acid) and
- Proteins (building block: amino acid).

1

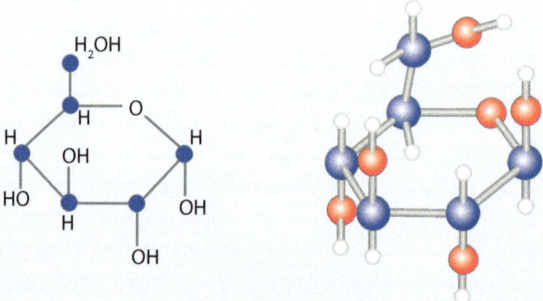

Structure of a molecule of dextrose (called glucose). A molecule of glucose consists of several atoms. Blue spheres represent the atom carbon (C), white spheres represent hydrogen (H) and red spheres represent oxygen (O). The arrangement is largely constant as a hexagon. The gray connecting lines are made of moving electrons.

Fig. 1.2 Structure of a dextrose molecule (called glucose)

At this point, let's take a closer look at the example of dextrose (■ Fig. 1.2). Dextrose, henceforth referred to as glucose, is a perfect chemical form of energy, as we can absorb glucose into every cell and break it down there. But what do we do with it and why?

With the help of inhaled oxygen in the air, this hexagonal glucose molecule is completely broken down into carbon dioxide (CO_2) and water (H_2O) through many precisely defined degradation steps within a cell. This breakdown is called glycolysis (glucose = dextrose; and lysis from lysis [λύσις] = dissolution)—so glucose dissolution.

The breakdown of glucose produces energy in the form of a universally valid "energy currency" in the body, called ATP. ATP stands for adenosine triphosphate, a molecule with 10 carbon atoms, 16 hydrogen atoms, 5 nitrogen atoms, 13 oxygen atoms, and 3 phosphorus atoms (hence "tri"). The mints of ATP are the mitochondria. Mitochondria were once independent bacteria (protobacteria) that were absorbed by other bacteria at some point. A symbiosis of protobacterium and bacterium emerged, and this coexistence has proven itself in the course of evolutionary history, as it still exists in our body cells today.

With ATP, you can pay almost anywhere, which is why ATP production is constantly and everywhere running. Unlike in real life, where there are only a few mints (in Germany: Berlin, Hamburg, Karlsruhe, Munich, and Stuttgart), each cell has many such "mints". Tissues with high turnover need more ATP and therefore have more mitochondria. ATP is produced during the breakdown of the three basic nutrients, namely carbohydrates (building block: e.g. glucose), fats (building block: fatty acid), and proteins (building block: amino acid). ■ Figure 1.3 shows the paths in a cell.

So when we talk about energy in the body, molecules like glucose and ATP are behind it. Molecules like glucose, fatty acids or amino acids can actually flow relatively freely in the blood, so from a purely physical point of view, one can also speak of an "energy flow" or better an energy flux. This is how—and only how—

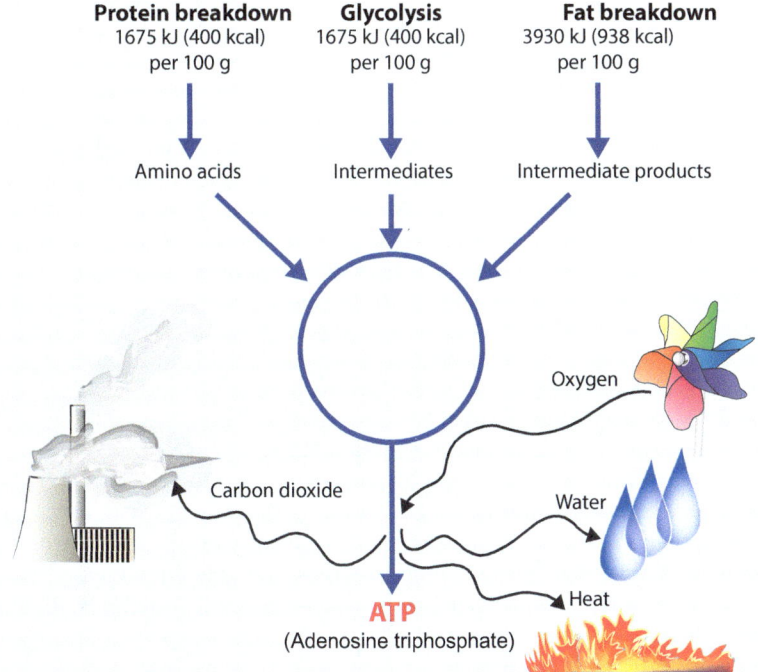

Breakdown of the main energy sources in food within a cell. Starting with proteins, glucose (glycolysis) and fats, degradation processes are initiated in the cell that lead to the breakdown of complex energy sources and ultimately result in the formation of ATP and heat. ATP is the central energy currency. ATP is produced in the coin factory of the "mitochondrion" (not shown). Oxygen is needed for this, and carbon dioxide, water and heat are produced in the process (see directions of the black arrows). Incidentally, energy can only be produced from glucose without oxygen.

◘ Fig. 1.3   Breakdown of the main energy-rich substrates in food within a cell

energy is distributed in the body (we will talk about distribution later) (see Infobox "Explanation").

Explanation: Energy Flow in the Human Body

For example, one could calculate the number of glucose molecules per vessel cross-section and duration, so there could be a unit like number of molecules per square meter per second. Since these molecules contain a lot of energy, the unit can also be converted into joules per square meter per second: so energy per square meter and second.

In physics, there is also the concept of energy flow, where the transfer of energy between different technical or natural systems is meant.

- Energy can then flow from place A to place B per unit of time and then has the unit joule per second.
- Energy can flow through a cross-section and then has the unit joule per square meter.

1

— Energy can flow through a cross-section per unit of time and then has the unit joule per square meter per second, which is the same unit as for the flow in the vessel.

Energy flows in the sense of vitalism are not meant at all. And when "the energy flux along the spine is blocked", it is unclear what is meant.

By the way, nothing comparable flows in nerves, as no substance is transported from A to B during the spread of excitation in the nerve. Only the activation state on/off is propagated along the nerve fiber from A to B. This is achieved by movement of ions through the membrane, which is an energy-consuming process.

The human body is an open system in terms of energy, and one wonders where it would be open. We saw that oxygen can be absorbed from the breathing air (open lung), or that glucose can be absorbed with food (open intestine). We also saw that when glucose is broken down, carbon dioxide (CO_2, the greenhouse gas) and water (H_2O) are produced, which also leave the body via the breath (open lung) and urine (open kidney). So there is nothing like energy conservation in the sense of a thermos flask. This "openness" has the great disadvantage that infectious germs can enter and exit, and infections and activation of the immune system are an extremely important topic in this book.

1.6 CAEN ("Controllable Amount of Energy") or How Much Energy Does the Body Need?

In the amount of substance called 1 mol of glucose, there are about 6×10^{23} such hexagonal molecules of glucose (◘ Fig. 1.2). This is an unimaginably large number of hexagons with 23 zeros after the six: 600,000,000,000,000,000,000,000 (600 trillion). But this mole of glucose weighs only 180 grams, and this amount of substance contains 2803 kilojoules or 2803×1000 joules (670 kilocalories), about as much as in a bar of chocolate.

A person of average size with a sedentary life style needs 10,000 kilojoules (or 2388 kilocalories) per day. If we wanted to cover the entire requirement with glucose, we would have to eat about 642 grams of pure glucose or 2183 trillion of these described hexagons. At this point, we want to simplify the units a bit because they will appear so often in the text. For the kilojoule we simply write "kJ" and for the kilocalorie we write "kcal". In addition, kJ is always mentioned first and then the kcal in brackets. Joule is the physically correct unit, which is deposited for the energy in the International System of Units in Paris. As already indicated, James Joule has thus won his dispute with Robert Mayer, otherwise it would be called Kilomayer today.

If you were a cyclist in the Tour de France and wanted to conquer the Col du Tourmalet in the French Pyrenees, you would need up to 30,000 kJ (7165 kcal) per day. A long-distance runner who would run all day like a marathon runner would need 140,000 kJ (33,432 kcal). Pheidippides—the first marathon runner around 490 BC—ran about 40 km and not all day, and according to legend he died of exhaustion. However, the story of death from exhaustion is doubted, as a trained runner should have easily covered this distance even then.

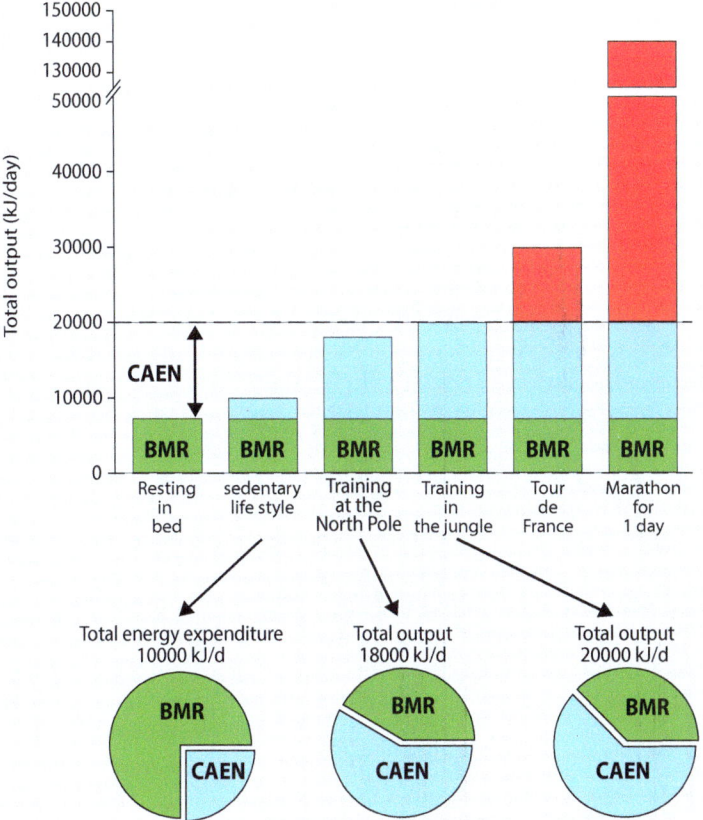

Comparison of energy expenditure per day in healthy people during various activities (4.1868 kJ = 1 kcal). When resting in bed, you need a basic requirement (called BMR in the figure) for the functioning of the cells etc., which in the example here is around 7,500 kJ (1791 kcal) (first green column from the left). Even a sedentary life style requires slightly more energy per day (small light blue area in the second column from the left and corresponding pie chart).This light blue area is usually referred to as activity-related energy expenditure because it is associated with physical activity. When training at the North Pole or in the jungle, the activity-related energy expenditure increases significantly (third and fourth columns from the left and corresponding pie charts). The basal metabolic rate (BMR) cannot be negotiated between the organs. In contrast, the CAEN ("controllable amount of energy") is the negotiable energy expenditure, which is distributed between the organs through control and steering mechanisms. Further explanations in the text.

Abbreviations:
CAEN = controllable amount of energy
BMR = basal metabolic rate

■ **Fig. 1.4** Comparison of energy expenditures per day in healthy humans at various activities (4,1868 kJ = 1 kcal)

A soldier in jungle training needs 20,000 kJ (4777 kcal) per day and a soldier in the Arctic ice 18,000 kJ (4299 kcal). The conditions are shown in ■ Fig. 1.4. There is also an important dashed line shown, which runs through the 20,000 kJ (4777 kcal). What is the significance of this line?

The 20,000 kJ (4777 kcal) mark is an important boundary line, indicating how much energy can be maximally absorbed per day through the intestine in the form

1

of solid energy-rich food and energy-rich liquids. It is also referred to as the *intestinal absorptive capacity*.

If a Tour de France cyclist consumes 30,000 kJ (7165 kcal) on a working day, he cannot cover these energy expenditures exclusively through food and fluid intake due to the intestinal absorption limit. He is, so to speak, starving, even though he is consuming huge amounts of glucose hexagons. When you starve, you lose weight. Since a cyclist's weight is based on muscles and bones, there is a risk that the cyclist will break down his urgently needed muscles. That's why cyclists repeatedly take smaller intermediate actions (short time trials on flat terrain or uphill) or proper rest days for regeneration, which is nothing more than eating, drinking, and resting a lot.

The FAZ titled an article on February 15, 2016, "The Big Feast" and it continues "Outsmarting the feeling of satiety: Shoveling, gulping, stuffing… Please do not disturb! During the carnivore feeding, the Tour de France riders prefer to be alone." Yes, it is not so easy to stuff in 20,000 kJ (4777 kcal), especially not when you only weigh 65 kg and are 185 cm tall (common for these cyclists).

We have learned that we need 10,000 kJ (2388 kcal) for sedentary activity (see above: Infobox "Explanation"), and that 20,000 kJ (4777 kcal) represent the intestinal absorptive capacity per day. However, if we were lying in bed, it would be cozy warm and we would not lose any energy through heat, if we would be more or less constantly dozing thoughtlessly and doing absolutely nothing, we would not need 10,000 kJ (2388 kcal) but only about 7500 kJ (1791 kcal). So even if you do nothing and don't freeze, you still need quite a lot of energy. This basal metabolic rate is needed for the elementary supply of the organs and muscles, which then also produce heat on the occasion. Even if you think the organs and muscles are doing nothing, they are doing quite a lot. The organs extract nutrients from the blood: hexagons (glucose), the fat molecules as fatty acids, or the protein building blocks as amino acids.

Explanation: Kilocalorie and Kilojoule

One kilocalorie is 4.1868 kilojoules or vice versa: 1 kilojoule is 0.2388 kilocalories. When examples of kJ values are mentioned in this book, they refer to a body height of about 180 cm and a body weight of 85 kg. Corresponding tables for other body measurements can be found in the standard work by Black et al.

Under the conditions in the warm bed, the cells draw their basic needs from the flowing blood. So there is a fundamental energy flow to the various organs, which is also little negotiable. Because without this energy flow, a cell in an organ or even the whole organ dies. From a certain basal amount of energy, the organs do not negotiate with each other, because each organ is dependent on the functioning of the other.

In a human body, a lot of energy is illustrated with the intestinal absorptive capacity, so 20,000 kJ (4777 kcal). Little energy is illustrated with the basal metabolic rate that is not negotiated, so about 7500 kJ (1791 kcal). The difference between the maximum intestinal absorptive capacity and the basal metabolic rate, which is roughly 20,000 kJ − 7500 kJ = 12,500 kJ (2986 kcal), can be negotiated. We call it here the *controllable amount of energy* (CAEN) (this is the black double arrow in Fig. 1.4).

But which organ needs the most energy?

1.7 The Big Three

An organ is, for example, the brain, the liver, the heart, or the kidney. An organ system is all muscles taken together or also the immune system, which are composed of many individual muscle packages or immune cells and can be located in many different places in the body. Immune cells are primarily located in the bone marrow, in the spleen, in the many lymph nodes, and in the thymus. But immune cells are also very common in the skin or in the intestinal wall, in the liver, and in the lungs. Therefore, we also speak of a skin immune system, an intestinal immune system, or a lung immune system, because the described "openness" of the system is particularly blatant there. There, the immune cells serve the local tissue surveillance, and they protect us from infections, but also from cancer diseases. They recognize foreign pathogens or degenerated tumor cells to kill them.

How much energy do these organs and organ systems now need? Table 1.1 gives an overview.

When in Table 1.1 "*includes the immune system*" is written, it means that the number mentioned would actually have to be reduced by the energy amount of the local immune system. The immune system consists of various cell types that are present in these various organs at a certain time, quasi on patrol or in fixed camps (= lymph nodes), to detect and neutralize infectious agents or other foreign material. These cells constantly need energy.

If you now look at the numbers for the organ systems and the organs in Table 1.1 and consider the slightly increased numbers due to the local immune system, then three organs or organ systems are particularly distinguished as main consumers: **Muscles, Brain** and **Immune System**. We can casually call these three organs or organ systems "*The Big Three*".

"*The Big Three*" is a reference to many such trios such as the three major film festivals in Cannes, Venice and Berlin, the three largest car brands in Germany (VW/Audi/Porsche, BMW and Mercedes-Benz) or the three largest economic powers in Europe (Germany, France and Great Britain). The significance of "*The Big Three*" will be examined more closely later with regard to the controllable or negotiable amount of energy, the CAEN. But first, we want to deal with the storage of energy in the body, because after all, the energy that can be released from stores is also negotiable.

1.8 Why We Store Energy—Fever, Tour de France and Newborns

A key characteristic of the human body from an energy perspective is the openness of the system: energy can be absorbed and released. Energy is absorbed in the form of heat over the surface or through energy-rich food and liquid. It is released over the surface as heat, as kinetic energy during physical activity, or in urine/stool in the form of chemical energy that is still present in the excreted energy-rich substrates.

1

◘ Table 1.1 Total energy expenditure in various situations and energy expenditure of organs and organ systems in a human during a day (180 cm and 85 kg)

Organ/Organ system	Energy expenditure per day kJ/d (kcal/d)
Resting human without activity (basal metabolic rate, non-negotiable)	7500 (1791)
Intake limit in the intestine	20,000 (4777)
Negotiable amount of energy (CAEN = intestinal absorptive capacity – basal metabolic rate)	12,500 (2986)
Human in usual sedentary activity	10,000 (2388)
Cyclist in the Tour de France	30,000 (7164)
Iron-Man participant at the World Championship in Kailua-Kona, Hawaii	37,500 (8957)
Marathon runner (extrapolated to the day; cannot be achieved in reality)	140,000 (33,432)
Additional expenditure in relation to the usual during pregnancy (all 266 days)	126,000 (30,095)
Additional expenditure in relation to the usual on average during pregnancy per day	474 (113)
Additional expenditure in relation to the usual during breastfeeding (all 180 days)	320,000 (76,431)
Additional expenditure in relation to the usual on average during breastfeeding per day	1778 (425)
Expenditure for growth and weight gain of 1 kg body weight	25,000 (5971)
Human after minor surgeries	11,000 (2627)
Human with multiple bone fractures (polytrauma)	up to 13,000 (3104)
Human with sepsis	15,000 (3582)
Human with burn injuries	≥20,000 (4776)
Sum of all muscles at rest*	2500++ (597++)
Brain at rest** (not such a big difference between rest and high activity)	2000 (478)
Immune system in all organs at rest*	1600++ (382++)
Mildly to moderately activated immune system in all organs*	2100++ (501++)
Liver (includes the liver immune system)	1600 (382)
Heart muscle at rest*	1100++ (263++)
Gastrointestinal tract (includes the gut immune system; excluding liver, kidneys, spleen)	1000 (239)
Kidneys	600 (143)
Spleen (red and white blood cells)	480 (115)
Lungs (includes the lung immune system)	400 (96)
Skin (includes the skin immune system)	100 (24)

* The two plus signs "++" mean: Especially the skeletal muscles and the heart muscle, but also the immune system, can consume much more energy when activated
** The brain, even with high activity, increases energy expenditure little, but constantly needs a lot of energy
Abbreviations: kcal = kilocalorie; kJ = kilojoule (10,000 kJ = 2388 kcal)
"*The Big Three*" are highlighted in bold

Imagine a summer vacation on the Mediterranean, where you bask in the sun or lie under the sunshade. On such days at 25–32 degrees Celsius, much less energy is needed to maintain the constant body temperature than on winter days at 0 degrees Celsius. In the zone between 25 and 32 degrees Celsius, our own heat production is at its lowest. From 32 degrees Celsius upwards, more energy is needed because you expend significantly more when sweating. Of the consumed energy mentioned in ◘ Table 1.1, about 85% goes into heat production, with which we maintain the constant body temperature of 37 degrees Celsius.

In addition to this, the remaining 15% is for various service functions of the entire body. Service functions include:

- Pumping blood through the vessels (heart work),
- Adjusting vessel diameter (vascular muscle work),
- Breathing (diaphragm muscle work),
- Stomach and intestinal movements (muscle work),
- Substance excretion in the kidney and intestine (ion pumps),
- Nerve functions (ion pumps),
- Muscular work and
- Cellular functions such as ion and substance transport across cell walls and formation of cell components such as cell proteins, cell walls or renewal of the genetic substance DNA and various other factors with which the cells communicate with each other (hormones etc.).

This list is not complete, but it gives a rough picture of why we consume energy at all. It is heated (85%), and a permanent service (15%) is maintained.

If we increase the body temperature by only 1 degree Celsius during fever, we need 13% more energy. If our body temperature during fever increased by 3 degrees Celsius from 37 to 40 degrees over a whole day, we would need 3900 kJ (931 kcal) more on that day in relation to the normal situation of 10,000 kJ (2388) with a sedentary life style, i.e. 13,900 kJ (3319 kcal). The figures show that heat production alone accounts for a large part of energy expenditure. As naked mammals, we are not well insulated and therefore lose heat more easily over the body surface. A Bernese Mountain Dog, which wears its black and white fur coat even in high summer and pants friendly, is better insulated.

As we have seen with the cyclist in the Tour de France, however, muscle work can also lead to a sudden increase in energy requirements (from the usual 10,000 kJ with a sedentary life style to 30,000 kJ per day). So there are various possibilities for a sudden increase in energy expenditure. In ◘ Table 1.1 the values are marked with "++" where particularly quickly and much additional energy can be expended. Here, the immune system and the musculature are primarily to be mentioned (including heart muscle). The brain needs little more extra energy with increased mental effort. However, the brain is crucial for the increase in energy expenditure through skeletal muscles, because after all, the brain decides whether to cycle over the Col du Tourmalet or run 42 km in the marathon.

A third possibility for a rapid increase in energy expenditure are large repair and growth processes, which is why burns, pregnancy and body growth are mentioned in ◘ Table 1.1 for comparison. In cows, milk production is a factor of high energy consumption, and glucose is consumed above all. Glucose is converted into lactose,

1

and this, along with fatty acids, is a crucial energy component of milk. Modern dairy cows like the German Holstein Black and White with high milk production therefore constantly experience hypoglycemia because glucose in the form of lactose disappears in the milk in the udder. But also breastfeeding mothers need a lot of extra energy, as shown in ◘ Table 1.1.

So if we need energy quickly for any special activities, it is extremely valuable to have a certain amount constantly available. This is particularly relevant when the immune system is activated by an infection, as energy intake can collapse massively then. Do you remember the last real flu over a period of a week? Did you have a great interest in taking your favorite foods or drinks or anything at all? No, of course not, because in such situations we switch on an emergency system that draws on the stored energy, which can lead to rapid weight loss. We will come back to this absolutely essential information several times in the book.

Even with very active mental or physical activity (which is often linked), energy intake is restricted, and one has to access stored forms of energy until one is again in a rest phase. With long mental/physical activity, the rest phases are short, and food intake is insufficient. Only the reserves help, if you have any.

A beautiful example of energy storage is given by human newborns. Compared to other creatures of similar maturity, they store a lot of energy in adipose tissue. Human babies are among the "fattest creatures" at the time of birth in relation to size, and this is still true up to a year after birth. It is assumed that this energy storage was vital when we still came into contact with the pathogens of the outside world under much worse hygienic conditions. It is quite clear that fat babies are better protected because they can mobilize more energy for the active immune system in an emergency. That's probably why we find really round babies so adorable, and probably why mothers and grandmothers love babies who eat and drink particularly well.

So how much energy can we store?

1.9 How Much Energy Do We and Our Ancestor Australopithecus Store?

The energy storage is enormous, for example, a man of today with 86 kg body weight can store about 550,000 kJ (approx. 130,000 kcal) or the energy of 216 bars of chocolate. ◘ Table 1.2 gives an overview of the energy storage of our male ancestors, the modern man and for comparison of today's domestic pig and chicken. It can be seen that our distant ancestors such as *Australopithecus* (3–4 million years ago) could only store half the amount of today's quantity. However, the *Australopithecines* were also only about half as heavy. Nevertheless, this amount of energy is not unlimited, and if no more energy is available or can be taken in, one dies.

How long would the energy stores last if one cannot intake energy in the form of food or energy-rich liquids? When does one die from emaciation?

To answer this, we make the following considerations: If one takes the "stored energy" from ◘ Table 1.2 and divides it by the daily energy consumption, as it roughly occurs during a flu infection, then one obtains the duration until all energy

1.9 · How Much Energy Do We and Our Ancestor Australopithecus Store?

19

1

■ **Table 1.2** Energy storage and emaciation time in our ancestors, in modern humans, in the domestic pig, and in the chicken

Our ancestors and modern human and for comparison two domestic animals	Time interval (Years)	Weight (kg)	Stored Energy (kJ)	Emaciation time* (Days)
Our ancestors and modern human				
Australopithecus afarensis	3.9–3.0 Mio.	45	275,502	27.9
Homo erectus	1.8 Mio.–200,000	66	485,500	40.6
Homo neanderthalensis	250,000–30,000	70	509,846	41.4
Homo sapiens	250,000–1900	65	377,130	31.8
Homo sapiens (Female)	today (USA)	74	545,052	43.1
Homo sapiens (Male)	today (USA)	86	558,908	41.0
Domestic animals today				
Pig (today)	65 Mio. years distance**	100	754,611	58.0
Chicken (today)	300 Mio. years distance**	3.7	21,177	18.3

* The duration until all stored energy is consumed is based on an energy consumption similar to a flu infection. Furthermore, it is assumed in the calculation that no energy is taken in the form of food or liquid
** The distance refers to the time interval to our last common ancestor in the common evolutionary history. Humans and pigs had their last common ancestor about 65 million years ago. After that, we have developed quite differently

reserves are consumed, i.e., until death in case of a flu infection. We want to call this time until death the "emaciation time".

However, this calculation assumes that no energy in the form of food or liquid is consumed during the disease leading to emaciation. Since one can intake little energy during the severe phase of a flu, for example, this is at least true for the first days of illness. From day 5 to day 10 it gets increasingly better, while severe infectious diseases can have a long course of 14 to 21 days. It can be seen that a modern human has an emaciation time of 41 to 43 days. Our ancestors, due to their lighter body structure, had a significantly shorter emaciation time of only 28 days until complete energy consumption and death. The modern domestic pig, which has large amounts of muscles and fat, can rely on 58 days without energy intake, and the modern chicken on respectable 18 days (■ Table 1.2).

The energy is mainly stored in the adipose tissue in the form of fatty acids and in the muscles in the form of protein (amino acids). ■ Figure 1.5 shows the energy stores of the human body. We can also store energy in the form of glucose in the liver and kidney (as starch), but this amount is small compared to the fat in the adipose tissue and the protein in the muscles. In the adipose tissue, a person with a body weight of 86 kg can store about 500,000 kJ (120,000 kcal or 200 bars of chocolate) and in the muscles 50,000 kJ (12,000 kcal or 16 bars of chocolate).

We have seen that a lot of energy is needed during a flu infection. Similarly, we need a lot of energy when we work physically or are active in sports. It now becomes clear that under certain conditions one has to rely on stored energy. We call

1

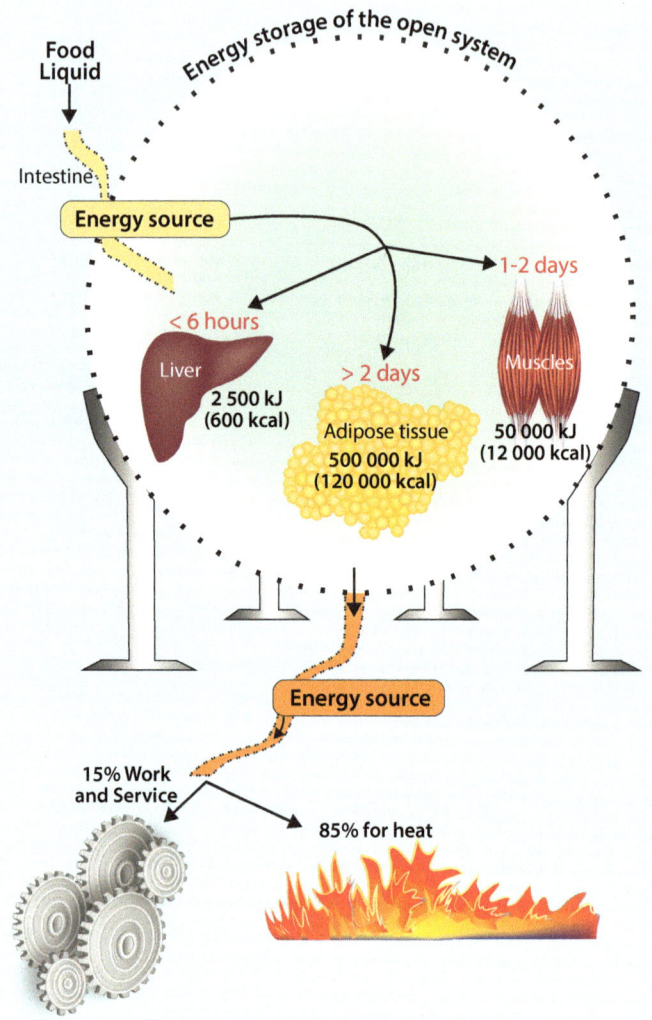

Energy stores in the human body. The liver stores starch (a form of glucose), fat tissue stores fatty acids, and muscles store starch and mainly protein. Below the organs or organ systems, the amount of energy and above it a time is indicated in red. The liver provides the fastest energy for less than 6 hours, the muscles provide energy for about 1-2 days, and then the energy supply from the fat tissue starts after day 2. From day 3 onwards, energy comes only from adipose tissue during starvation. Ultimately, most of the energy is "burned out the window" in the form of heat. Only 15% goes into services and light physical activity (see text).

▪ **Fig. 1.5**   Energy stores in the human body

the human body and that of *Australopithecus* energetically open, which is why it needs energy stores to survive.

Before we get to the regulation of energy allocation to the various organs, we need to clarify which type of energy-rich substrate (glucose, fatty acids, amino acids) the three most consuming organs—the brain, the muscles, and the immune system—need. "The Big Three" are picky.

1.10 Sweet Tooth—Brain, Muscles, and Immune System

Glucose is the favorite of all organs and organ systems. It's like in real life, because there it's also the case: "Most people like sweets." Surprisingly, however, some claim "Sugar is poison for the body." The truth is, too much sugar is unfavorable, but sugar or glucose cannot be a poison, as this substance is urgently needed and is present everywhere in the body.

Organs love sugar because it can be quickly and profitably converted into the ATP coin. Moreover, it can be easily stored in the form of animal starch (= interconnected hexagons) in the liver, kidneys, and muscles. Then, glucose can also be broken down (glycolysis) when there is no oxygen (which is not the case for fatty acids). This can become important, for example, during inflammatory reactions in the tissue or during intense physical work in the muscle, because there is often an undersupply of oxygen. Glucose is also important in all those tissues that normally have to cope with little oxygen (cartilage tissue, ligament tissue). Moreover, the glucose ingested in the diet is absorbed in the intestine faster than the other energy-rich substrates (fatty acids, proteins/amino acids). These are great advantages of glucose, which is why it is so central to the big energy business and the food industry.

For example, the brain mainly relies on the energy supply from glucose. The brain can also use a substitute meal of ketones, but that's not fun. Because when the brain gets this substitute meal, we don't feel quite right. The brain needs sugar. So, we are almost like an addict, sugar-addicted.

Muscles can process glucose, fatty acids, and amino acids, and they are therefore not as picky as the brain. The cells of our immune system are also not picky, as they can use all energy-rich substrates. However, it is the case that muscles and the immune system also prefer glucose, because they often have to work without oxygen. In ◘ Fig. 1.3 it was shown that oxygen is needed to produce the ATP coin. Under special conditions, however, glucose can also be used for the oxygen-free production of the ATP coin. This makes glucose a piece of gold under oxygen-poor conditions.

What's special about the provision of glucose is also the fact that when muscle proteins are broken down, those amino acids are released that can be converted into glucose in the liver. So, when the muscle provides stored energy-rich substrates in the form of amino acids, glucose is made from them. Also, breakdown products of glycolysis, as they occur in the various organs, can be regenerated to glucose in the liver. However, for the regeneration of a hexagon glucose you have to put down five ATP coins, because regeneration is expensive. In general, the liver can convert the energy-rich substrates into each other, which is why the liver could also be called a "switchboard," because it does not appear as a large energy storage (◘ Fig. 1.5). In the switchboard, the building blocks arrive and are then converted into another building block and returned to the blood, which all costs a lot of energy.

Now we are at a point where we can talk about the regulation of energy flows. We start with foraging before we discuss energy storage.

1.11 Food Search Prior to Energy Storage

If one can store and expend energy, there must also be a regulated build-up and breakdown of energy stores and an energy flow to the consuming organ. The energy should transfer into the bloodstream in the form of glucose, fatty acids from adipose tissue, and amino acids from protein-rich muscles, and then be taken up by that organ or organ system that most urgently needs the energy at the given time. It should be noted in advance that fundamentally different messenger substances are important for energy storage and energy release, as their significance is also fundamentally different.

The messenger substances come from the world of nerves (called neurotransmitters), hormones from glands, and cytokines (cytokines are primarily messenger substances from immune cells, but also from other cells). ◘ Figure 1.6 describes these messenger substances in more detail. These messenger substances can exert the necessary long-distance and short-distance effects. Nerves exert long-distance effects through an excitation that is propagated along a nerve pathway (e.g., from the brain to the adipose tissue [Fig. 1.6] or from the brain to the pancreas, etc.). Hormones and cytokines enter the bloodstream and thus cause long-distance effects (◘ Fig. 1.6). Hormones and cytokines can also exert long-distance effects by influencing the brain, for example (◘ Fig. 1.6).

At the top of energy storage is the brain with its eating and satiety centers. If a deficiency is signaled, the eating center becomes active, and we go in search of food.

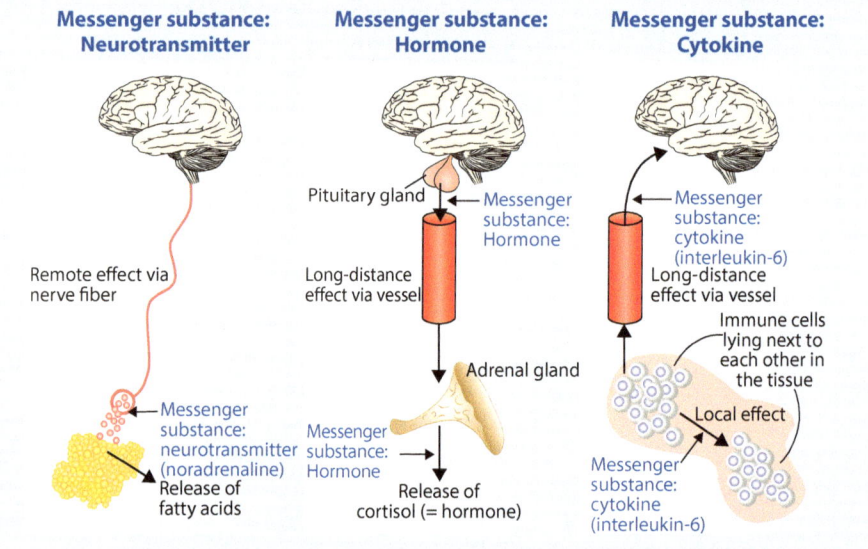

Messenger substances in the human body - short- and long-range effects. From left to right, the three categories of messenger substances are shown here: neurotransmitters from nerve fibers, hormones from endocrine glands and cytokines from immune cells. Neurotransmitters can produce short-range effects between cells in close proximity and long-range effects between organs and organ systems. The long-distance effect via nerve fibers is considerably faster than via hormones or cytokines.

◘ **Fig. 1.6** Messenger substances in the human body—short and long-distance effects

Since the refrigerator or supermarket is not far away these days, we expend little energy in the search for food. In contrast, imagine the hunting Eskimo in Arctic Canada, who consumes much more energy in the search for food. In contrast, we, largely sedentary people, take in more energy than we actually need. Consequently, we also store too much.

Under natural conditions, the hunt for edible food is a rather energy-consuming process. For example, a group of Stone Age hunting Pygmies in Africa was observed and it was found that on three randomly selected consecutive days, slightly more energy was expended for hunting and searching than was taken in by consuming the hunted food. Hunters cannot afford such imbalances for too long. It shows that hunting for edible food under natural conditions is very energy-consuming. The hunt then yields about as much as one needs daily under conditions of higher activity.

But what are the decisive mechanisms for energy storage?

1.12 Neuronal Factors and Hormones of Energy Storage

Under favorable conditions after food intake, without physical activity and in a sufficiently warm environment, energy is stored. Since the gastrointestinal tract is essential during food intake, the main organizer of the gastrointestinal tract—the **vagus nerve**—is very important for the uptake of energy-rich substrates and for storage. The vagus, as it is also briefly called, receives its work signals from the brain, and it also sends signals to the brain. The vagus promotes intestinal activity and digestion, and it is also crucial for the release of insulin from the pancreas.

Insulin is the main storage hormone (◨ Fig. 1.7). Insulin is primarily known because it is used as a medication in diabetics. In diabetics, it works by removing

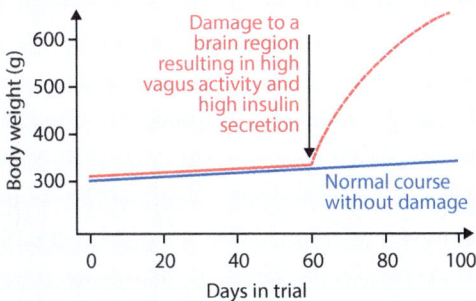

Importance of the vagus nerve and insulin for body weight. Here, a center in the brain of rats was damaged, resulting in significantly higher activity of the vagus nerve. With the increased activity of the vagus nerve, a significantly higher insulin secretion and a dramatic increase in weight were observed (red curve compared to the blue curve).

◨ **Fig. 1.7** Significance of the vagus nerve and insulin for body weight glucose from the bloodstream to store it in muscle and adipose tissue. In this way, insulin performs the function of a storage hormone and a medication, and it lowers blood sugar levels. Insulin can also remove fatty acids from the blood and store them in adipose tissue and muscle. Insulin is the great remover of energy-rich substrates from the flowing blood.

By now, other storage hormones are known. Namely, those hormones that promote muscle growth and therefore increase the storage of protein, glucose, and fatty acids in the muscle. First and foremost is the **testosterone**, the male sex hormone. Testosterone and all so-called male sex hormones (androgens; from *andros*, gr. man) promote muscle and bone growth. A professional bodybuilder typically takes male sex hormones to increase muscle mass, but also increases the risk of prostate cancer and the like. The androgens also increase the storage fat in the abdominal area, so that fatty acids can be stored there more intensively. Androgens are produced in the testes and in the adrenal gland (see Infobox "Explanation").

Explanation: Role of the Adrenal Glands

The adrenal glands are glands that sit like caps on both kidneys. They are each the size of an apricot and produce various hormones that are released into the blood stream.

One distinguishes the adrenal **cortex**, from which cortisol and androgens originate. In the adrenal cortex, an important hormone for blood pressure regulation is also produced.

Furthermore, one distinguishes the adrenal **medulla**, which is surrounded by the cortex (similar to the apricot kernel by the apricot flesh). In the adrenal medulla, adrenaline is produced. Adrenaline is the number 1 stress hormone released into the blood stream.

The brain is the supreme master of the adrenal gland, which hormonally controls the adrenal cortex via the pituitary gland (◘ Fig. 1.6) and the adrenal medulla via the sympathetic nervous system. The adrenal cortex and adrenal medulla belong to the stress system.

Female sex hormones, the **estrogens**, are storage hormones insofar as they are responsible for the typical fat distribution and accumulation in women and for bone growth. Estrogens are produced in the young woman of reproductive age in the ovaries. In menopausal women, estrogens are produced from androgens of the adrenal gland (see Infobox "Explanation"). You read correctly! Estrogens always originate from androgens. They are formed by a special enzyme from androgens like testosterone. However, estrogens cannot be converted back into androgens. This is a one-way street. In older women, androgens are converted into estrogens in many tissues. So, in menopause, estrogens are produced locally—as needed—from the precursors (the androgens from the adrenal gland).

Last but not least, **Vitamin D** is also a storage hormone as it promotes muscle and bone growth. If the bone has been listed as a storage here, this has an important meaning, as the bone is the largest storage for calcium, phosphate and magnesium. These chemical elements are absolutely necessary for many cell functions, which is why a storage must be present. During our evolutionary history, our ancestors left the sea for land about 350 million years ago. In the sea, there was always enough calcium and phosphate, as these elements are present in high amounts in seawater. When moving to land, a storage of chemical elements was necessary because one was not constantly flooded by seawater. The bone is an incredibly large reservoir for calcium, phosphate, and magnesium.

■ Figure 1.8 summarizes the regulation of energy storage.

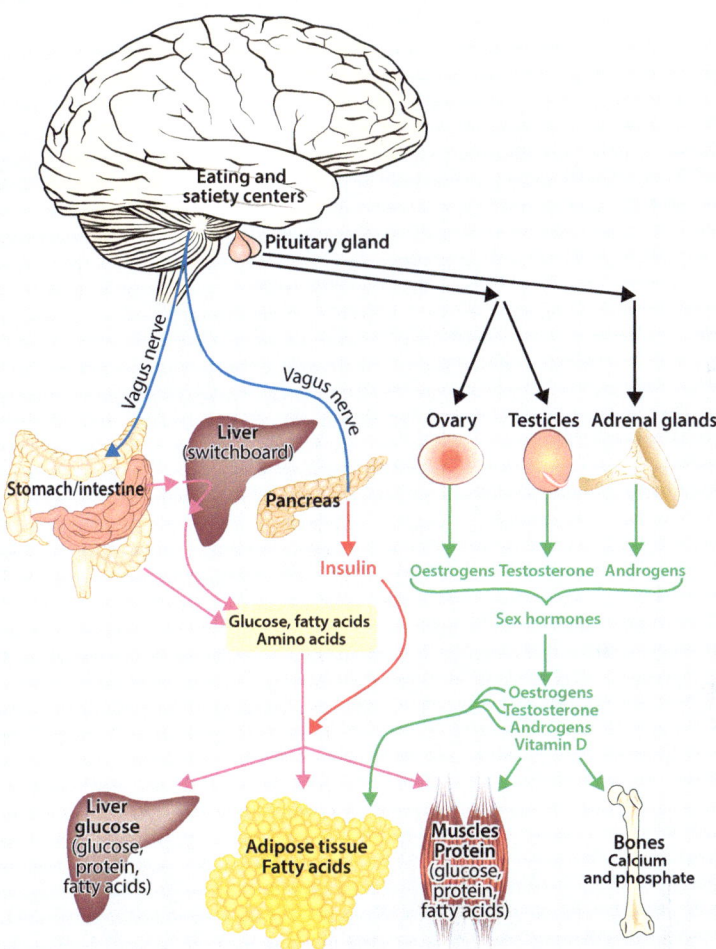

Regulation of energy storage in the human body. Energy sources such as glucose, fatty acids and amino acids are absorbed in the gastrointestinal tract and partly made transportable by the liver so that they can be transported in the blood on container ships. The most important storage factor is the hormone insulin from the pancreas. It is responsible for ensuring that glucose and fatty acids are absorbed in the liver, fat tissue and muscle. The sex hormones and vitamin D are jointly responsible for growth and thus for the size of the storage sites (muscle, fat tissue and bone). This is where the amino acids, fatty acids, calcium and phosphate are incorporated. The arrows from the pituitary gland represent hormones that originate in the brain and have a controlling effect in the periphery. The vagus nerve also originates from the brain and plays a crucial role in the release of insulin. It is important to mention that under these normal storage conditions, messenger substances of the immune system hardly play a role (they are not mentioned separately).

■ **Fig. 1.8** Regulation of energy storage in the human body

1

1.13   A Little Lesson on Stress Hormones

We have already learned about the adrenal gland in the infobox explanation (see above), here comes more. If we now consider the essential factors for the release of energy-rich substrates from the stores, we recognize fundamentally different players. These are mainly the sympathetic nervous system with the neurotransmitters **Adrenaline** and its brother **Noradrenaline**, the **Cortisol** from the adrenal gland and **pro-inflammatory cytokines** of the immune system.

The three hormones noradrenaline, adrenaline and cortisol are stress hormones, which are released upon activation of the stress system. Cytokines are usually released in the area of inflammation during inflammatory stress. Before we get to the regulation of energy release, we first want to examine the four factors more closely in terms of terminology. After that, the individual factors will be considered in relation to energy release.

We usually only talk about adrenaline and mean the hormone that is released during stress and gives us a powerful kick. Adrenaline is also the emergency drug for cardiac arrest. Noradrenaline is hardly mentioned, although it is at least as important as adrenaline. Noradrenaline is used similarly to adrenaline in the case of cardiovascular shock, for example in severe sepsis.

Both hormones are biologically highly active. Noradrenaline is found mainly in the endings of sympathetic nerves (◘ Fig. 1.6) and adrenaline mainly in cells of the adrenal medulla. Noradrenaline is thus released near the nerve ending, while adrenaline enters the bloodstream and thus produces a remote effect. Both areas—the nerve endings and the adrenal medulla—belong to the sympathetic nervous system.

The activation of these two sympathetic areas is started in the brain (release within seconds to minutes). For example, a psychologically stressful event like a near car accident leads to activation, and a shiver runs through us from head to toe. An encounter with a lion in the savannah causes the same effect. For experienced !Kung warriors[1] in the Kalahari, it might not be quite as dramatic.

In addition to the two stress hormones adrenaline and noradrenaline, there is also the hormone cortisone of the adrenal gland. The layman says cortisone and means the "therapy with cortisone", but the body's own biologically active hormone is called cortisol. In fact, cortisone is an inactive form of the biologically active cortisol, which is why one should pay particular attention to the correct use of these terms. The use of the word cortisone has historical reasons, because the discoverers of cortisone actually treated a patient with joint inflammation (arthritis) with the biologically inactive form of this hormone.

Fortunately, the biologically inactive cortisone is converted into biologically active cortisol in the body (e.g., in the liver), and so the doctors achieved an excellent therapeutic success when using cortisone, for which they were awarded the Nobel Prize for Medicine in 1950. For the rest of the text in this book, the term cortisol will be used to correctly denote the biologically active form of the hormone. Cortisol is produced in the adrenal cortex and quickly released during stressful events (within 15 minutes).

---

1   The exclamation mark is a phonetic sign in the click language.

Here you already notice that the adrenal gland with its medulla and its cortex is a central organ in fight, flight or stress. The adrenal gland releases the stress hormones adrenaline and cortisol into the bloodstream, whereas the sympathetic nerves release noradrenaline in the direct vicinity of the nerve ending. All three messengers are at the center of our fight-and-flight equipment.

1.14 A Brief Lesson on Immune Messengers

Finally, we come to the immune messengers—the so-called cytokines of the immune system (■ Fig. 1.6; cyto = cell, kine from kinisi = move). Cytokines are often called pro-inflammatory because they are fundamentally involved in the activation of inflammation. This is particularly the case at the beginning of infections or when there is a risk of infection from a wound. Among others, TNF (= tumor necrosis factor), interleukin-1, and interleukin-6 are pro-inflammatory cytokines.

There is a huge number of cytokines, and it is impossible to discuss them all. Cytokines are immune messengers that mediate effects between closely adjacent cells of the immune system, i.e., they move something between cells. Typically, cytokines have little long-distance effect, as they are intended to act only very locally. This applies, for example, to TNF and interleukin-1.

However, some cytokines of the immune cells are also proper long-distance messengers, such as interleukin-6 (■ Fig. 1.6). Interleukin-6 is a stable factor that can circulate in the bloodstream for a long time and thus have an effect elsewhere (■ Fig. 1.6). For example, interleukin-6 from immune cells in the spleen can stimulate the distant pituitary gland and the distant adrenal glands to produce cortisol and adrenaline, at least temporarily. Thus, one could also call interleukin-6 the hormone of the inflammation focus.

Cytokines are usually found in larger quantities in the blood only when there is an inflammation focus somewhere. By the way, these cytokines also lead to an inflammation constellation, which we can recognize by an increased erythrocyte sedimentation rate (abbreviated ESR) or an increased level of C-reactive protein (CRP).

1.15 Stress Hormones and Cytokines Release Energy

Finally, we come to the factors for the release of energy from the stores, after we have mentioned the corresponding storage factors above. Noradrenaline is crucial for the release of fatty acids from the large fat tissue store. There, the sympathetic nerve fibers are in close proximity to fat cells, so that the release of fatty acids is activated when noradrenaline is released (■ Fig. 1.6).

Adrenaline can also stimulate the release of fatty acids from the fat store, but it does this primarily in abdominal fat and less in peripheral fat tissue (this is the task of local sympathetic nerve fibers and noradrenaline). However, abdominal fat is also the fastest to break down, as one can notice with great joy and happiness after short periods of hunger. The first 1–2 kg are quickly lost when dieting.

1

In addition to the two messenger substances of the sympathetic nervous system, cortisol can also stimulate fat breakdown in normal amounts. This shows that all three stress hormones release fatty acids from the fat tissue store. However, cortisol can deposit fat in unusual places (face, neck) when present in higher amounts, resulting in the typical "cortisone" appearance as a side-effect of therapy. However, this special case plays hardly any role in energy storage.

Cytokines like TNF are also involved in the release of fatty acids from the fat tissue, as they inhibit the effect of the storage hormone insulin. In addition, cytokines like interleukin-6, in the sense of long-distance effect, activate the sympathetic nervous system and thus release noradrenaline and adrenaline. Furthermore, many cytokines activate the pituitary gland, which in turn stimulates the release of cortisol. In this way, cytokines can indirectly break down fat stores.

The situation is similar with the mobilization of glucose, which is stimulated by the three stress hormones. This glucose is stored in the form of starch in the liver and muscle. However, the reserves in the liver only last for about 6 hours (◘ Fig. 1.5), and the muscles do not release the glucose at all, because they only want to access it themselves (with regard to glucose, the muscle is selfish). Therefore, the glucose store in the liver is rather small as an energy store when compared to the fat stores in the fat tissue. However, all three stress hormones cause a new formation of glucose from precursors, which has already been described as regeneration of glucose and takes place in the liver (gluconeogenesis).

In addition to its influence on fat release and glucose regeneration, cortisol can also promote muscle breakdown and thus leads to the release of important amino acids, which can also be incorporated into glucose regeneration. Some cytokines like TNF also have this function.

Furthermore, noradrenaline, adrenaline, cortisol, and certain cytokines such as TNF, interleukin-1, and interleukin-6 are **bone-degrading** factors. This relationship is known in the case of cortisol, as bone degradation is a serious side effect of "cortisone therapy" with higher doses (this is called bone loss or osteopenia, e.g., in the treatment of patients with inflammatory rheumatic diseases).

In addition to the three most important stress hormones and the cytokines of the immune system, there are three more stress messengers that need to be briefly discussed here. The **growth hormone** from the pituitary gland increases glucose regeneration and fat breakdown, the **thyroid hormones** support norepinephrine and adrenaline, and the **RAA hormones** (see Infobox "Explanation") from the kidney and liver perform glucose release and bone degradation. All are on the side of energy release or bone degradation (release of calcium, magnesium, phosphate).

At this point, a question may be allowed: Wouldn't it make sense if the energy-releasing factors would inhibit the effect of the energy-storing factors and vice versa? This is indeed the case, as noradrenaline, adrenaline, cortisol, the cytokines such as TNF, growth hormone, thyroid hormones, and the RAA hormones all inhibit the effect of insulin, the main storage hormone. They essentially nullify the effect of insulin directly at the cell by making the cell resistant to insulin. Then the uptake of glucose or fatty acids into the storage cell no longer works. These energy-rich substrates are then available to other organs. In addition, the activation of the sympathetic nervous system (norepinephrine/adrenaline) is accompanied by an inhibition of the vagus, so that significant intervention can also be achieved in this way, because then the insulin secretion is inhibited. Nothing is stored anymore because the storage hormone insulin is missing.

Explanation: RAA hormones (Renin, Angiotensin, Aldosterone)

The main task of the RAA hormones is in blood pressure regulation. One might wonder why blood pressure regulation has anything to do with acute stress. Well, if you encounter a lion in the savannah, it makes a lot of sense for blood pressure to rise. Increased blood pressure enhances performance because it boosts blood flow to the brain and muscles. Then you can fight better or run away faster. The other extreme is very low blood pressure, as in circulatory shock, a state of complete performance loss.

During stressful events, blood pressure must be high, and energy-rich substrates must be provided. If the systems are thus coupled, it makes sense. The coupling is perfect insofar as the sympathetic nervous system with its messengers noradrenaline and adrenaline stimulates the RAA hormone system. Both, the sympathetic nervous system and the RAA hormone system, thus raise blood pressure and ensure the provision of circulating energy-rich substrates.

By the way, the increase in blood pressure works as follows: The RAA hormone system and the sympathetic nervous system raise blood pressure by reducing the excretion of water in the kidney and constricting the vessels. The water thus remains in the constricted vascular system, and this increases blood pressure.

Also, cytokines such as TNF and interleukin-1, which are released in an inflammation site, inhibit the activity of the vagus nerve and insulin. These are therefore good prerequisites for stopping all storage processes when energy is needed in the short term.

Isn't it fascinating how these stress hormones all together release energy from the stores, simultaneously increase blood pressure, and also degrade bone and muscle? Without a doubt, these hormones—noradrenaline, adrenaline, cortisol, growth hormone, thyroid hormones, and the RAA hormones—really fire up our body. They are the partners in sports, in combat, in bleeding, in emergencies, in injuries, in encounters with lions, in stress of any kind.

These hormones must be incredibly good. They are the shot of adrenaline junkies who plunge into the depths with a rope (bungee jumping), jump over abysses with a motorcycle, parachute (parachuting), jump with skis over rock slopes (freeride skiing), plummet from high rock edges into the valley in wing suits (base jumping), do handstands on the carrying cables of the Golden Gate Bridge (handstanding), slide down narrow gorges on the wet seat of their pants (canyoning), and much more. It's not just adrenaline, the other hormones help too.

On the other hand, the pro-inflammatory cytokines are only released very specifically in the case of inflammation or inflammatory stress, but they can also circulate in the bloodstream and have a remote effect, and they have many similar effects to the stress hormones, namely energy release, muscle degradation and bone degradation. However, they are definitely not junkie factors, because their release is associated with a feeling of illness, and that is not at all cheerful. This is a big

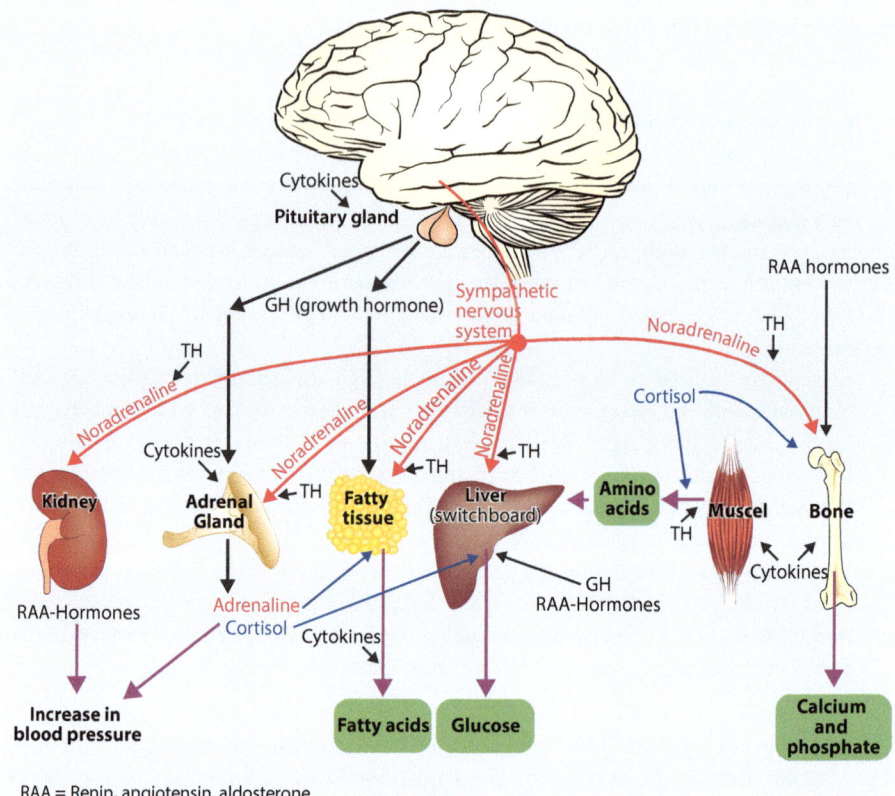

RAA = Renin, angiotensin, aldosterone
TH = thyroid hormone
GH = growth hormone

Regulation of energy release in the human body. The sympathetic nervous system with the main messenger substances noradrenaline and adrenaline and the adrenal gland with cortisol are the central factors in the provision of energy (fatty acids from fat tissue, glucose from the liver and amino acids from the muscle; highlighted in green), bone resorption and increased blood pressure. They receive help from the growth hormone (GH), the thyroid hormones (TH), the RAA hormones (= renin, angiotensin, aldosterone) and the cytokines of the immune system, which in turn cause the release of energy at various points and break down bone and muscle. Thyroid hormones help noradrenaline or adrenaline wherever they have an effect (arrow with TH). Arrows generally indicate beneficial activity (arrows on bone and muscle indicate degradation). Cytokines include, for example, the pro-inflammatory TNF, interleukin-1 and interleukin-6.

Fig. 1.9   Regulation of energy release in the human body

difference between the stress hormones on the one hand and the cytokines on the other. Why this is so different will be discussed in more detail later.

Figure 1.9 shows the regulation of energy release, and Table 1.3 summarizes energy storage and energy release again. Always return to Table 1.3, Figs. 1.8 and 1.9, and you will understand large parts of the book.

1.16 A New Look at the CAEN ("Controllable Amount of Energy")

We want to end this chapter with a consideration of the CAEN. It has been shown that the basal metabolic rate is non-negotiable (in the above example in ◘ Table 1.1 it was 7500 kJ [1791 kcal]), and that only the CAEN of a maximum of 12,500 kJ (2986 kcal) can be negotiated between the organs (◘ Fig. 1.4). The energy release factors are used for negotiation (◘ Fig. 1.9 and ◘ Table 1.3). If there are three major consumers, "*The Big Three*", one can assume that these three main consumers—brain, muscles, immune system—are significantly involved in the negotiation. Depending on which consumers need the energy, they will intervene accordingly to claim the CAEN for themselves.

◘ **Table 1.3** Regulation of energy storage and energy release in the human body

	Fat tissue (Fatty acids)	Muscles (Amino acids)	Liver (Glucose)	Bones (Calcium, Phosphate)	Blood pressure
Energy storage					
Vagus nerve	Intake		Intake		
Insulin	Intake	Intake	Intake		
Testosterone*		Growth		Growth	
Androgens*		Growth		Growth	
Estrogens*	Intake	Intake		Growth	
Vitamin D		Growth		Growth	
Energy release					
Sympathetic nervous system (Noradrenaline/Adrenaline)#	Release	Release	Release	Release	Increase
Cortisol#	Release	Release	Release	Release	Increase
Growth hormone#	Release	Release	Release		Increase
Thyroid hormones#	Release	Release	Release	Release	Increase
RAA hormones#			Release	Release	Increase
Cytokines (TNF)#	Release	Release		Release	Decrease
Cytokines (Interleukin-6)##	Release##	--	Release##	Release##	
Danger signals###	Release	Release		Release	

* These factors promote insulin in its action
# These factors inhibit the action of insulin
Interleukin-6 stimulates the pituitary gland and the sympathetic nervous system, resulting indirectly in the release of energy-rich substrates (effect only short-term)
Danger signals are released during cell decay and are recognized by immune cells, which then produce cytokines and thus indirectly release energy-rich substrates (not shown in ◘ Fig. 1.9)

In ▪ Fig. 1.9 and ▪ Table 1.3 we recognize many hormones influenced by the brain and the sympathetic nervous system with its neurotransmitters among the energy release factors. In addition, we also recognize the cytokines (for example TNF, interleukin-1 and interleukin-6) and the cellular danger signals as important factors for energy release. Interestingly, the muscle can also produce interleukin-6, and so it should also be involved in energy release. However, voluntary muscle work (including heart work) is mainly dependent on the brain, so the active muscle itself does not have to take care of the release of energy stores if the brain already takes over this job with the appropriate hormones and the sympathetic nervous system. Brain and skeletal muscles build a psychomotor unit, and the brain is hierarchically above the muscles.

In the next chapter we will go into more detail about who really are the major negotiating partners for the distribution of the CAEN. It will be seen that this question can be clarified with simple considerations from the field of evolutionary medicine. The negotiating partners must necessarily influence many fates in the body in health and, as we will see later, also in disease.

A sentence at the end of this chapter: Even if Chap. 1 was a bit difficult, don't let it deter you from continuing to read! It will now get easier and easier, because in Chap. 1 you were equipped with the tools to understand the energy regulation of our body. Things repeat themselves, and you quickly get a picture of the whole. The illustrations of Chap. 1 with the corresponding references will be referred to again and again throughout the book.

You have taken the biggest hurdle.

In a nutshell

- In an isolated system, energy remains constant. A *perpetual motion machine* does not exist.
- There are various forms of energy (e.g., thermal energy, kinetic energy, chemical energy) that can be converted into each other.
- From an energy perspective, the human body is an open system that absorbs and releases thermal energy and chemical energy.
- Three crucial nutrients are absorbed as energy-rich substrates: carbohydrates (e.g., glucose), fats (fatty acids), and proteins (amino acid).
- The breakdown of energy-rich substrates takes place in every cell, and the energy coin ATP (adenosine triphosphate) is mainly produced in the coin factory named mitochondrion.
- In a sedentary way of life, we need about 10,000 kJ (2388 kcal) per day, while resting in bed we need a basal metabolic rate of about 7500 kJ (1791 kcal) per day, and the absorption limit in the intestine is 20,000 kJ (4777 kcal) per day.
- This results in the negotiable, controllable energy, briefly CAEN, to 20,000 kJ (4777 kcal) minus 7500 kJ (1791 kcal) = 12,500 kJ (2986 kcal). CAEN can be negotiated between the organs.
- "*The Big Three*" or the big three energy consumers are muscles, brain, and immune system.
- When "*The Big Three*" are very active, hardly any food is taken in, which is why energy stores must be present to cover the demand by redistribution from the stores.
- The emaciation time in case of illness and food stoppage is about 6 weeks.

- The main energy storage is the adipose tissue followed by the muscles; the liver is a switchboard that converts energy-rich substrates into each other and regenerates glucose from degradation products, which also consumes energy.
- Energy storage factors are:
  - Vagus nerve,
  - Insulin,
  - Testosterone and other androgens,
  - Estrogens and Vitamin D.
- Energy release factors are:
  - sympathetic nervous system with noradrenaline and adrenaline,
  - Cortisol,
  - Growth hormone,
  - Thyroid hormones,
  - the blood pressure stabilizing RAA hormones (= Renin, Angiotensin, Aldosterone) and
  - many cytokines of the immune system.
- Energy release factors are responsible for the controlled distribution of the CAEN ("controllable amount of energy").
- The main consumers—brain, muscles, immune system—are partners in the negotiation of the CAEN.

References

Black AE, Coward WA, Cole TJ, Prentice AM (1996) Human energy expenditure in affluent societies: an analysis of 574 doubly-labelled water measurements. Eur J Clin Nutr 50: 72–92

Blaxter K (1989) Energy metabolism in animals and man. Cambridge University Press, Cambridge

Caneva KL (1993) Robert Mayer and the conservation of energy. Princeton University Press, Princeton

Hirschberger J (2007) Die Geschichte der Philosophie in 2 Bänden. Komet Verlag, Köln

King BM, Carpenter RG, Stamoutsos BA, Frohman LA, Grossman SP (1978) Hyperphagia and obesity following ventromedial hypothalamic lesions in rats with subdiaphragmatic vagotomy. Physiol Behav 20:643–651

Margulis L (1999) Die andere Evolution. Spektrum Akademischer Verlag, Heidelberg

Meulders M, Garey L (2010) Helmholtz – from enlightenment to neuroscience. Massachusetts Institute of Technology Press, Cambridge

Planck M (1887) Das Princip der Erhaltung der Energie. B.G.Teubner Verlag, Leipzig

Straub RH (2015) The origin of chronic inflammatory systemic diseases and their sequelae. Academic, San Diego

Wenzl A (1951) Hans Driesch – Persönlichkeit und Bedeutung für Biologie und Philosophie von heute. Verlag Reinhardt, München

Yamauchi T, Sato H (2000) Nutritional status, activity pattern, and dietary intake among the Baka hunter-gatherers in the village camps in cameroon. Afr Study Mongr 21:67–82

Evolutionary Medicine

Contents

2.1   Darwin, Wallace & Co.—Simultaneity of a Discovery – 36

2.2   Darwinian Evolution—Species and Selection – 37

2.3   Darwinian Evolution—Modern Additions – 38

2.4   Chickens from Behind – 39

2.5   Founder Effect in Canada, Lactose Intolerance and Fat Babies – 42

2.6   The Selfish Brain – 44

2.7   The Selfish Immune System – 46

2.8   When Two Fight … – 47

References – 49

2

2.1 Darwin, Wallace & Co.—Simultaneity of a Discovery

Charles Darwin was born on February 12, 1809, in Shrewsbury, England. After primary school, he studied medicine at the University of Edinburgh. However, his father soon noticed that his son had no interest in medicine, but rather spent his time with natural history and natural science studies and was more interested in the writings of his grandfather Erasmus Darwin—a natural philosopher.

So he sent him to Christ's College in Cambridge, and Charles had to pursue a career as a clergyman. However, his academic performance was not good enough to achieve these goals. Meanwhile, he was much more interested in natural philosophical matters, and he completed his studies with a *Bachelor of Art* in Theology in 1831—with this level of education, he could not become a clergyman. During this time, he began his famous beetle collection. Stimulated by the American research trip of Alexander von Humboldt from 1799–1804, Charles Darwin now wanted to contribute to natural history studies himself.

Fortunately, he had cast his net wide and early, and his botany professor John Henslow arranged for him to be employed as a naturalist on the HMS Beagle (HMS = His Majesty's ship), which set sail on December 27, 1831, for a nearly five-year journey. This trip, with stops in the Galapagos Islands and Australia, was a source of new insights for Charles Darwin, which earned him a reputation as an English naturalist during the journey itself.

His father organized private wealth and thus helped him to a financially worry-free life as a scientist. Charles Darwin spent many years working on his records and sorting the collection he had brought with him. From the notebooks, it is clear that he had already incorporated elements of his theory of evolution in 1837 and 1838, which would become so significant 20 years later, but had not yet published them. If one now asks why Charles Darwin published these findings only so many years later—not until 1859—there are several answers.

He certainly suffered from a chronic disease, the nature of which remains unclear to us today due to a lack of knowledge. He had several bouts that often prevented him from doing his work. After marrying his first cousin, Emma Wedgwood, in 1839, they had ten children between 1839 and 1856, and three of the children died at a young age. This included his dearly loved Anne Elizabeth, who died at the age of 10 from an infectious disease. These, in some respects, sorrowful paternal duties may have partly hindered him. Furthermore, he felt that the foundations of his theory needed to be substantiated by additional observations. But the most significant obstacle was the fact that he saw his own new considerations as a risk because they had to lead to a fundamental change in theological views—namely the creation dogma from the first book of Moses (Genesis). He wrote: "It feels like I'm confessing to a murder"—the murder of the act of creation.

Ultimately, in June 1858–20 years after the Beagle voyage—a manuscript sent to him by Alfred Russel Wallace, which outlined the principles of natural selection, stimulated him. Alfred Russel Wallace (1823–1913) is now considered an equal originator of the early form of the theory of evolution. He himself conducted extensive studies in the Amazon region and the Malaysian archipelago. The boundary line between different ecozones in Asia and Australia is named after him (*Wallace Line*).

The ecozones divide the earth into different biogeographical areas with different ecological characteristics. Anyone who has seen a kangaroo, a wombat, a platypus, a koala, the laughing kookaburra, and other curious, unknown animals elsewhere in the wild in Australia can understand how Wallace came up with the idea of a boundary line and consequently natural selection.

Wallace's manuscript was then published simultaneously with a hitherto unpublished work by Charles Darwin from 1844 in the form of a reading before the English Carl von Linnean Society in the absence of both authors (July 1, 1858). Perhaps they were afraid of immediate criticism, although interestingly, the usual discussion did not develop immediately after the reading. Wallace's writing now stimulated Darwin to complete his elaborate book *On the Origin of Species* within the next year and a half. It was published on November 22, 1859.

So what does the theory of evolution say?

2.2 Darwinian Evolution—Species and Selection

In the following, we want to describe the concept of species and the Darwinian theory of evolution in more detail, and we will see at the end what enormous significance it has gained for medicine. But what is actually the concept of species (□ Fig. 2.1).

Darwin himself struggled with the concept of species, and the definition is not addressed in his books. The concept of species for Darwin is probably best described as a reproductive community, so he used the biological definition. This biological definition has been particularly favored from the second half of the twentieth century (by Theodosius Dobzhansky and Ernst Mayr). Ernst Mayr wrote:

"A species is a reproductive community of populations and is isolated from other reproductive communities in terms of reproduction. The species occupies a specific niche in nature."

The theory of evolution is attributed to several people who contributed between 1858 and the mid-twentieth century. In the following text, the decisive elements of the theory are highlighted in bold. Darwin's first book already contains the following decisive principles of the early form of the theory:[1]

- There is an **excess of offspring**. Despite this constant surplus, population sizes do not change (the number of individuals remains stable). This results in a corresponding reduction of the excess of offspring.
- There is inherited variability (**heritability** and **variation**).
- As a result, individuals better adapted to their respective environment have a greater probability of surviving the competition (**natural selection**). We say of a species that still exists today that it has been **positively selected**. This means that the species or a trait of a living being (e.g., a red comb) has undergone positive selection after many generations, so it is still there. The trait was positively selected. In contrast, all species that no longer exist today and are extinct have undergone negative selection, they were **negatively selected**.

---

1   In the German words of Gerhard Heberer in the afterword to the German edition of the Darwin book in the Reclam publishing house from (1963).

Kingdom (Animals)

Phylum (Vertebrates)

Class (Mammals)

Order (Primates)

Family (Apes)

Genus (Homo)

Species (Homo sapiens)

Systematics in the animal kingdom with a special focus on the species "Homo sapiens." Homo sapiens belongs to the family of apes and to the genus Homo. The species is defined on the basis of morphological criteria, biological functions (reproduction as a criterion: only representatives of a species can produce fertile offspring) or phylogenetic affiliation. According to the latter definition, a species begins after a phylogenetic species split and ends after extinction or with a new species split. All definitions have advantages and disadvantages and lead to different classifications. The systematics go back to *Carl von Linné (Linnæus)*.

◘ Fig. 2.1   Systematics in the animal kingdom with a special focus on the species "Homo sapiens"

— This selection of better adapted variants progressively leads to a change of the species (**evolution**).

The phrase "*Survival of the Fittest*" is not from Darwin himself, but was coined by the social philosopher Herbert Spencer (1864). However, Darwin also used this term in later editions of his first book. Although the essential elements of the theory of evolution were recorded in this first book, additions have been made over time that make up the modern form of the theory of evolution.

2.3 Darwinian Evolution—Modern Additions

After Darwin's death, more precise ideas about heredity soon emerged, first formulated in 1866 by Gregor Mendel, then forgotten for three decades and finally rediscovered around 1900. They are also known as Mendel's laws of inheritance.

The following points were added in the course of time, which from about 1940 onwards are referred to as the "modern synthesis of evolutionary theory:

- The inheritable material is subject to individual, spontaneously arisen variations despite high constancy (**Mutation**, Hugo de Vries, 1901).
- The inheritable material is located on the chromosomes in the cell nucleus (**Gene** or **Genes** define the trait or traits), and mutations can occur in all orders of magnitude (Thomas Hunt Morgan, 1907–1926).
- Variation is created during reproduction by exchanging alternative forms of the same gene (so-called alleles) and by rearranging genetic material, where whole pieces of the genetic substance (DNA) can be moved back and forth and reassembled (**Recombination**, also T.H. Morgan and his working group).
- Studying entire populations allows to study the frequencies of traits and thus of associated genes in a reproductive community (**Population genetics**, many scientists,[2] between 1910 and 1940).
- On the basis of these population genetic considerations, insights into **Isolation, Migration, Genetic drift** and **Founder effect** emerged, which form the basis of speciation. Isolation is recognized as reproductive isolation (no offspring can be produced, although originally the same species was present), ecological isolation (ecological niche) and geographical isolation (spatial separation of populations of the same species). Genetic drift is a random change in allele frequency in a population's gene pool (can happen, for example, by dividing into smaller subpopulations). The founder effect is important when colonizing a new area with a small population, as a founding father or mother could have brought a piece of hereditary information that is disproportionately increased (an example is mentioned in the next but one section).
- Natural selection tests the newly emerged and is the dominant factor of evolution, leading to the adaptation (**Adaptation**) of individual organisms of a population. Adaptation refers to adaptation to environmental conditions.
- **Macroevolution** (i.e., the development of large type differences above the species level, such as genus, family, order and above, ◘ Fig. 2.1) and **Microevolution** (i.e., the development of small differences within the species, e.g., between ethnic groups) can both be explained as a continuum from microevolution to macroevolution through mutations and selection. There are no logical or biological leaps (example: development of the eye).

2.4 Chickens from Behind

At this point, we leave the strict scientific aspect of evolutionary theory and clarify various things in simple words. Evolutionary theory is often misunderstood because we humans are goal-oriented. We remind ourselves every day anew that we have to accomplish this and that, perform this action at this and that time, want to achieve this or that in our lives, etc. We mainly project into the future and have little left for the past. We think in self-set goals and determine beforehand (*a priori*) how

---

2   Theodosius Dobzhansky, Sergej Četverikov, Ronald Fisher, John B.S. Haldane, Godfrey H. Hardy, Julian Huxley, Ernst Mayr, B. Rensch, George G Simpson, Wilhelm R. Weinberg, Sewall Wright, Nikolai Vavilov, George Yule and others (in alphabetical order).

we have achieved this and that afterwards (*a posteriori*). Humans are oriented in a "goal-finding way".

Due to the *a posteriori* considerations, evolutionary biology, unlike other branches of science, has a much harder time being understood by us humans. In physics, chemistry, engineering, etc., we think much more in terms of goals. An example from physics may illustrate this: If I accelerate a body of known mass, I need exactly this force (I aim for a force). In contrast, a special passive, less action-oriented, observing attitude is needed to view evolution as something that has already occurred. Ernst Mayr once wrote: "Adaptation to the environment … is an *a posteriori* result and not an *a priori* goal-finding."

So if you garden in your backyard with a goal-oriented approach, then with a bit of skill the desired flowers, shrubs and trees will grow. We think in categories of achievable things. But if you let everything grow, you will be amazed at the unexpected diversity. The wonder comes *a posteriori*, which can bring a lot of joy, especially when you have done little *a priori*.

Religions do not make it any easier for us at this point, as religions are goal-oriented. The Christian religion, for example, shapes the believer and sets the goal of eternal life for him. This requires certain behavior from the religious person, which is stipulated in the 10 Commandments and other places. We are shaped by this way of thinking because we learned about the act of creation of the world (Genesis) in religious education at a very early age.

This goal-oriented thinking can also be clearly seen in the so-called creationism, which is present in many places in the United States. The word creationism already says it: "Someone [God] created something." In many schools, evolutionary biological approaches are swept under the rug and creation myths are taught instead. Strict creationism defends the Bible and Genesis. According to this, the earth is only 6000 years old. Even in our schools—especially in the lower grades—the theory of evolution is neglected.

At this point, one should delve into the time periods of evolutionary history (◘ Table 2.1).

The periods mentioned in ◘ Table 2.1 are enormous, and it is difficult to estimate their magnitude. When we talk about common ancestors, they did not look like a human or the species mentioned in ◘ Table 2.1, because both—humans and respective species—have then evolved according to the time indicated in ◘ Table 2.1, without a goal, but as optimally adapted to the respective environmental conditions as possible.

So our common ancestor with chickens was neither a chicken nor a human, because both had 310 million years to undergo changes in shape, genes, biological functions, etc. during the course of evolution. So we did not descend from today's chickens.

Evolution must always be viewed from the back, and it does not have a direction from "simple" to "better". The currently present is not better than the past. Dinosaurs were present for 200 million years, but today only their descendants, such as chickens and crocodiles, are still alive. Are chickens and crocodiles better than dinosaurs? Silly question, right?

For example, when we think about the species mentioned in ◘ Fig. 2.1 today, we are looking back at the evolution that has taken place. And if an animal is excellently adapted to environmental conditions, then this is a view from the back,

⬛ **Table 2.1**   Distance between humans and the last common ancestors of the mentioned species in years

Species	Years before our era
Gorilla, Chimpanzee, Orangutan	6.5 million
Rat, Mouse, Rabbit	65 million
Pig, Cow, Goat, Horse	65 million
Dog, Cat	65 million
Dinosaur	310 million
Chicken, Snake, Crocodile, Turtle	310 million
Frog, Salamander	360 million
Coelacanth	400 million
Shark, Ray	420 million
Lamprey, Hagfish	460 million
Sea cucumber, Sea urchin, Sea squirt	515 million
Squid, Octopus, Snail, Lobster, Crab	530 million
Insects	530 million
Sponges	540 million
Plants, Fungi	more than 600 million
First bacteria (Stromatolites)	3.5 billion
Age of the Earth[*]	4.6 billion[*]

[*] The 6000 years from the Bible are comparatively short

i.e. after everything has already happened over millions of years. Evolution cannot be thought of in forward terms. So if modern humans exhibit a trait, this a-posteriori result is preceded by a long evolutionary process, the result is adaptation, and it can be assumed with great certainty that the trait is often also present in our direct ancestors, but also in much more distant ancestors of other species.

And that's actually the case! Even chickens, with whom we share the last common ancestor 310 million years ago, have an adrenal gland, a sympathetic nervous system, noradrenaline, interleukin-6 and overall a very similar energy regulation, as was presented in ▶ Chap. 1. If a good principle has proven itself, it is not simply abandoned. It means good adaptation to life on this earth. Take another look at the distance to the common ancestor with chickens in ⬛ Table 2.1. Thus, the energy regulation between chickens and humans has been quite—not in every detail—similar for 310 million years – e.g., the emaciation time (see ▶ Chap. 1, ⬛ Table 1.3 is relatively similar in humans and chickens).

Evolutionary medicine draws on such knowledge and thus generates an *ultimate* or fundamental framework that enriches biological and biomedical science. Medical science is almost always very goal-oriented with *proximate* objects that serve the immediate benefit of humans. Our current medical students are trained to be diagnostic and therapy machines that are supposed to achieve immediate, i.e. proximate financial—perhaps also humanitarian—successes. But in order to classify and understand the problems of humans and his current diseases in their basics, both the proximate **and** the ultimate view of the healthy and sick is needed. The proximate view focuses more on the individual and the ultimate view on the population or the species.

Although this ultimate starting point is self-evident in biology, human medicine has been and is very slow in recognizing this fundamental approach. The following section briefly introduces ultimate explanations, so that the significance of evolutionary medicine and its fundamental approach can be better assessed.

2.5 Founder Effect in Canada, Lactose Intolerance and Fat Babies

Imagine yourself in the sixteenth and seventeenth centuries in Canada. During these two centuries, already 125,000 Germans had emigrated to the area of today's USA. Not so many wanted to go to Canada, only about 1–5% of them. French people felt a stronger attraction to Canada, especially to the east (today's Quebec). But French immigrants were also found in the rest of North America. They called this land New France *(Nouvelle France)*. Commissioned by Louis XIV in 1608, a total of six settler families with a total of 31 people founded today's Quebec.

Among the early French settlers, there were probably a few people present who brought with them the genetic predisposition to rare diseases. This is particularly well known for a group of settlers from southern Normandy who emigrated to the Canadian region of Charlevoix-Saguenay around 1675. They brought with them a nervous disease that was and is rare in a large population in France, but was and is much more common in a newly founded small population. Thus, the rate of some rare diseases in French Canada is higher than in the French motherland or in Europe in general. This phenomenon is called the founder effect, as there were "disease founders" present among the approximately 2600 settlers who settled in this region.

In this way, migration can also lead to changes that influence the course of evolution. If we were not aware of this founder effect, we might look for completely different causes of disease that have nothing to do with the diseases (e.g., environmental influences, work influences, toxic influences, etc.). Therefore, recognizing the founder effect—an example from evolutionary medicine—helps the doctor to genetically explain diseases and thus to better treat them in the future.

Another example is lactose intolerance, which should be known to us because there are lactose-free milk and lactose-free foods in our supermarkets. About 90% of Germans do not buy these products, but people with lactose intolerance depend on them. In our intestine, there is a digestive enzyme called lactase (the corresponding gene plays the key role). Lactase has the task of splitting lactose (milk sugar) so that it can be absorbed in the intestine. Since all mammals and also humans depend on the early childhood supply of breast milk (at least it was like this for a long time), mammals and humans depend on lactase in these early years. After weaning, the activity of this enzyme is gradually shut down, so we react sensitively to lactose in the intestine (between the 2nd and 5th year of life). Because too much of the non-absorbable milk sugar causes bloating and diarrhea, and that's why the affected person goes to the doctor.

If we look at today's Europeans, about 90% of Central and Northern Europeans tolerate fresh milk well into old age. Also, 90% of Americans and Australians of European descent tolerate fresh milk in adulthood. In most regions of the world, especially in Asia and Africa and among the indigenous Australians and the indigenous people of North and South America, but also in the Mediterranean, it is quite different. In these regions, most people have lactose intolerance. If we consider the majority of the world's population (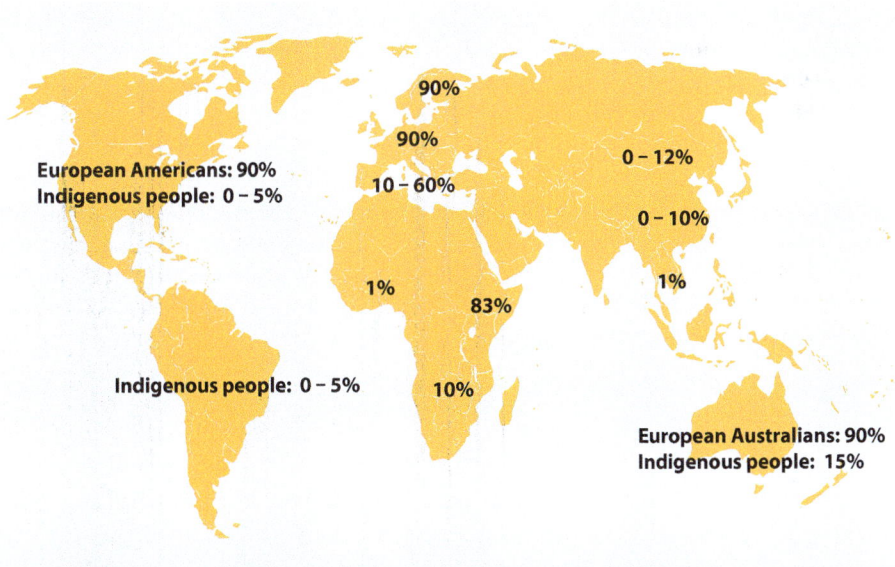 Fig. 2.2), then lactose intolerance is rather normal than pathological.

If the World Health Organization WHO classifies lactose intolerance as a metabolic disease, then 80% of the world's population have a gut disease, and that can't be right. People with lactose intolerance invented dairy dishes like kefir, yogurt, buttermilk, and curdled milk, where the manufacturing process with yeasts leads to digestion of the milk sugar. So the above-mentioned 80% of the world's population can very well consume dairy products in adulthood, just not fresh milk.

Today we know that tolerance towards milk was created by a genetic change in the gene of lactase about 10,500 years before our era. About 10,500 years before our era, milk-producing animals were domesticated by our human ancestors. This fit very well together because now in northern Europe with the new lactase in the intestine, the milk could be broken down. This genetic change led to milk tolerance in childhood and adulthood. Great mutation!

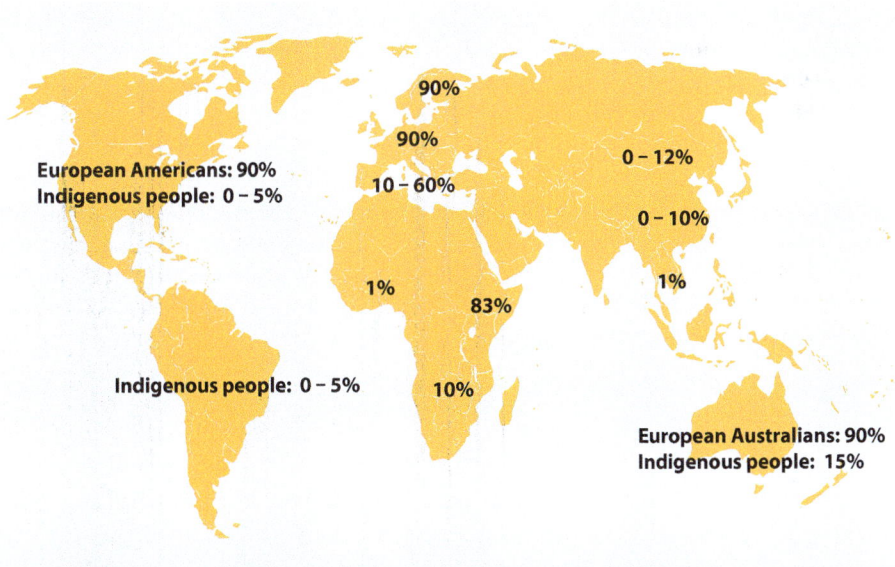

Distribution of milk tolerance on earth. The percentages indicate the frequency of people who tolerate fresh milk without any problems.

Fig. 2.2 Distribution of milk tolerance around the world

But not only Northern Europeans, but also East Africans, for example in Kenya, are capable of enjoying milk in adulthood. The Kenyans also have a change in the gene of lactase, which leads to milk tolerance. Interestingly, the genetic changes in Central and Northern Europeans are quite different from those in Kenyans, but the functional significance regarding good milk tolerance is identical. This principle is called convergent evolution. Convergent evolution leads to the same functionally significant trait, namely milk tolerance in adulthood, using different paths.

Because examples are so beautiful, a third insight is now presented, which also has great significance for today's people. In ▶ Chap. 1 "Energy and Body" it was shown that human babies, compared to most animals, have a body with a very high fat content. This fat store is useful when a baby becomes so sick from an infection that it can hardly take in any more food. Under these conditions, the baby shows typical *Sickness behavior* and lives off the stores, with fat stores being able to store the most energy.

Especially in small children up to the age of 6 with a not yet fully functioning immune system, this "fatty phase" is important, as the risk of infectious disease is highest. However, the "fatty phase" between 0 and 6 years is decisive for the formation of fat cells. During these early years, the number of fat cells is determined. If many fat cells are formed during this phase, they remain for a lifetime, and one can store fat excellently. For the Stone Age living human, this is very practical because he could create sufficient energy stores. This was particularly useful in case of infectious disease, but also in case of food shortage.

So, if there were one or more genetic changes (mutations) in our prehistory that led to an early childhood increase in the number of fat cells, and if this mutation was a survival advantage before puberty—i.e., before reproduction—then this advantageous mutation was gladly passed on to the next generation during reproduction. We then say: "The mutation remained in the gene pool" or "the mutation was retained throughout our evolutionary history." Since this early childhood predisposition to fat cells still exists in our children today, it must have been an important thing in our evolutionary history. If this excessive fat storage had been an obvious disadvantage in our newborn ancestors and therefore the fat children had not survived until the age of reproduction, then this phenomenon would no longer exist today. But since it still exists today, it must have been quite useful. Unfortunately, this also means that the potential for excessive fat storage is established early on, which causes us problems in adulthood.

2.6 The Selfish Brain

At this point in the book, you have acquired enough basic knowledge to now return to energy regulation. In ▶ Chap. 1 "Energy and Body" you learned that the main energy consumers in our body are the brain, the muscles, and the immune system. The energy stores are mainly created for these three organs. It was also hinted that *"The Big Three"* are probably the most important partners in the negotiation of controllable energy in the human body. The controllable energy—CAEN—is negotiable, and there are corresponding factors for this. The storage factors (◘ Fig. 1.8) and the release factors (■ Fig. 1.9) were discussed. ■ Table 1.3 provides an overview for both.

At this point in the book, we now link evolutionary medicine and energy regulation to get to know the main negotiating partners of the CAEN.

In a thought experiment, we put ourselves in the shoes of a Stone Age hunter who goes hunting with male peers in the savannah. One is tense, almost electrified. Especially the inexperienced ones are under high tension. One has dressed up in a warlike manner and painted one's face. They wear feathers on their heads to enlarge the body image and to look more dangerous. One carries a throwing spear and a stone knife. Everything has been well worked out, and the experienced ones prepared the inexperienced ones for the hunt. One feels the adrenaline, because a lion could break out of the thicket at any moment. According to Jared Diamond, the world-renowned evolutionary biologist, the Stone Age !Kung warriors from the Kalahari often exposed themselves to such situations. And then it actually happens—lions attack.

Who decides in this absolutely tense situation in our body? Who recognizes whether one should rather flee or fight? Who directs how we should cooperate with the hunting partners, and which methods are used? The brain, with its connections to the eye and ear and the rest of the body, is now the decisive control instance. No matter how we decide—whether flight or fight, the brain dominates the decision and in any case calls the voluntary muscles and the heart muscle to action.

This example clearly shows the close interlocking of the brain, voluntarily controllable muscles, and heart muscle. Every flight or fight action involves a high activity of the voluntary muscles and the heart muscle. And now one also understands why the muscles do not like to give up the stored energy (e.g., glucose, starch, or fatty acids). If muscles are to be prepared for the fight, then they must not give anything away during rest periods.

So, the brain and muscles are closely linked (it is a psychomotor unit). Under normal conditions, it is never the muscle that asks the brain to become active, but always the other way around. Due to its high importance in the struggle for survival, the brain occupies an absolutely central position in this fight and flight reaction. To put it pointedly, one can say that the brain dominates in fight and flight reactions because it is best for the survival of the individual.

Fight and flight responses can only last a short time, as they require very high energy expenditure. It was said: "Pheidippides—the first marathon runner around 490 BC—ran about 40 km and not all day, and according to legend, he died of exhaustion." Fight and flight responses cannot last long. In ■ Fig. 1.5 the energy stores in adipose tissue and muscle were discussed. These energy stores allow us to survive 41 days without food in the event of increased energy expenditure due to an infectious disease. We said: "The emaciation time in case of an infectious disease is about 41 days." However, if we were to expend as much in a day as a marathon runner (140,000 kJ [33,432 kcal] if he runs all day), then this time would theoretically be reduced to less than 4 days until death—not to mention that one would have an incredible need for sleep in between and therefore could not run a marathon for 4 days straight (the only exception might be Forrest Gump in the novel of the same name by Winston Groom, who could run forever and grew a long beard). One would surely die of exhaustion after 4 days.

2

In summary, it can be stated that the brain dominates the voluntary muscles and the heart during fight and flight and is therefore the highest authority for the distribution of CAEN. Thus, we have already found one of the two important regulators of CAEN. **We therefore call the brain selfish**, because it claims the CAEN for itself and the muscles dependent on it. The brain does not "ask" if any other organ has something to object. There simply isn't time to negotiate costly, as life is immediately threatened. The **selfishness of the brain** has been retained in our evolutionary history. Even in heat, cold, or when starving, the brain is the highest authority.

2.7 The Selfish Immune System

Now we turn to the consideration of the immune system, which has already been identified as a major consumer. We go back in evolutionary history to the time of the Neanderthals. If a Neanderthal inflicted a flesh wound on himself while playing with a spear, and this wound unfortunately became infected, he was already risking his life. Antibiotics have only existed since 1928, when Alexander Fleming discovered penicillin in England. It is not without reason that we vaccinate people against tetanus (lockjaw), who come to the emergency room with such flesh wounds. The Neanderthal had neither penicillin nor tetanus vaccination available. The Neanderthals were dependent on wound cleaning abilities and on immune cells, that is, the immune system. But the immune system needs energy.

Under favorable conditions, good wound cleaning, low number of pathogens, lesser pathogen danger, and decent immune system performance, the Neanderthal was soon healthy again. However, if a serious infection had developed, if the bacteria had penetrated deep, if an abscess had formed in the tissue, if this had caused a significant infection problem, then it could have become critical. The enormous energy consumption of the immune system could have led to death.

Abscesses are also a major danger for people living under Stone Age conditions today. Simple scratches can turn into serious local infections and mean death. Jared Diamond describes this situation in a book from 2012. There he came to the aid of a person in New Guinea who had been sick in a straw hut for many days because he had contracted a serious local infection from a scratch. The antibiotics he brought improved the patient's condition quickly. We want to make another example.

Consider the so-called Spanish Flu, which claimed at least 25 million lives worldwide between 1918 and 1920. Isn't it surprising in direct comparison that the just-ended First World War "only" claimed 10 million lives? People were firstly weakened after the end of the First World War, secondly the food reserves were low, thirdly the nutritional situation of the people was poor and the stored energy of each individual was at a low point.

Especially influenza can lead to a long duration of illness and severe emaciation, because secondary problems like bacterial pneumonia and similar can occur. In this energy deficiency, the sick person is confined to bed or in the case of the Neanderthals to the camp in the cave. Depending on the extent of the infection problem, a longer disease process can result here, which can lead to a critical strain on the energy reserves due to significantly reduced food intake because of *Sickness behavior*. And then it applies:

Without energy, no infection defense!

In both cases—in case of injury or flu—the immune system dominates. The immune system "does not ask" whether any other organ has something to object. Here, the other organs such as the brain, gastrointestinal tract (not the liver), voluntary muscles and heart muscle are shut down. There simply isn't time to negotiate costly, as life is immediately threatened. The selfishness of the immune system has been retained in our evolutionary history; this selfishness of the immune system is still present today. We therefore call this defense system the **selfish immune system**. Similar to the consideration of the brain, the immune system must now have the ability to claim the CAEN for itself.

2.8 When Two Fight …

If the brain and the immune system get in each other's way, it can become really critical, as both access the reserves. We can estimate such a situation where we have to perform a large workload for professional reasons, but at the same time are plagued by an infectious disease. These are very critical situations, as neither the brain nor the immune system function properly. Both influence each other in a negative way, they try to inhibit each other. Such an internal battle probably cannot be sustained for long.

In the case of increased work demands with simultaneous infection, the immune system usually wins according to the author's experience. That's why one of my colleagues recently said that the immune system must be even more selfish than the brain. Eventually, we end up in bed. The CAEN moves towards the immune system. The negotiations were negative for the brain. One could object here that they are ultimately positive for the brain, as this is the only way we can recover from infectious diseases and survive.

Examining the evolutionary history of humans has helped us to more easily imagine ourselves in a time of Stone Age hunters (which still exist today). It's not like today, when we stand in front of the supermarket shelf and the family doctor lives just around the corner. We can also draw further conclusions from examining evolutionary history. Just as it is for the Stone Age hunter, so it is for our direct ancestors (Homo), the great apes, all primates, mammals in general, vertebrates in a broader sense, and pretty much all animal species that fight, flee, and get sick from infections. Considering our evolutionary history, it becomes understandable that even more distant animals must exhibit similar mechanisms. Those who flee or fight need a recognizing brain and nervous system and muscles that do what the brain commands—fight or run away. Those who expose themselves to an infection need a recognizing immune system that overcomes the infectious agent or promotes wound healing. Since storage is limited, but fight/flight or immune defense cost a lot, the reaction must be time-limited. Most other organs not involved in this reaction must be reduced to their basal metabolic rate.

By the end of this section, it should hopefully be clear that we have two potentially conflicting negotiators regarding the CAEN:

- the selfish brain and
- the selfish immune system.

This basic consideration leads to an important regulatory principle: the brain and immune system must conduct negotiations as much as possible with their own means, so that the other can do little against it. This leads us directly to the consideration of the factors for energy release mentioned in ▣ Fig. 1.9.

In a nutshell

— Charles Darwin and Alfred Russel Wallace were instrumental in the first drafting of the theory of evolution in 1858.
— The first form of the theory of evolution incorporated:
   –surplus of offspring,
   –heritability,
   –variability,
   –natural selection (positive and negative selection),
   –adaptation changes species (evolution)
— The modern theory of evolution adds:
   –chromosome,
   –genes,
   –mutation,
   –recombination of genetic material;
   –population genetics defines rules and leads to ideas about isolation, migration, genetic drift and founder effects;
   –macro- and microevolution represent a continuum.
— A species is a reproductive community of populations and is isolated from other reproductive communities in terms of reproduction. The species occupies a specific niche in nature (Ernst Mayr).
— Humans think *a priori*, i.e., goal-oriented; however, evolution must be viewed from the back: *a posteriori*.
— Large periods of millions or even billions of years are difficult to grasp. With an average temporal distance between 2 consecutive generations of 20 years (today's human: 25 years), one gets 50,000 generations in a million years. We are separated from the first vertebrates by 460 million years (lamprey, hagfish).
— Humans did not descend from chickens. Chickens and humans had a common ancestor 310 million years ago, who was neither a chicken nor a human. Both had enough time to develop differently.
— Evolutionary medicine is a new field that contributes to the explanation of causes of diseases: for example, rare diseases in French Canada (e.g., Charlevoix-Saguenay), lactose intolerance without disease value, as well as fat storage, which existed in our ancestors and still exists in us.
— The brain is acutely active in fight and flight (muscle and heart are dependent on the brain, psychomotor unit). The immune system is acutely active in infection defense and wound healing. The energy consumed cannot be greater than the energy reserves. Thus, one can calculate the time of emaciation.
— There is a selfish brain and a selfish immune system. The organs not involved are reduced to basal energy need during acute activation.
— There are indeed *"The Big Three"* (brain, muscles, immune system), but regarding the negotiation of the CAEN ("controllable amount of energy") there are only

two egoists, as the brain controls the activity of the heart muscle and skeletal muscle.

— From an evolutionary medical perspective, the brain and immune system should be dominant and largely independent in the procurement of the CAEN. Therefore, separate factors of the brain or the immune system to claim energy from stores must exist.

References

Darwin C (1963) Die Entstehung der Arten. Reclam, Stuttgart

Diamond J (2012) The world until yesterday: what we can learn from traditional societies. Viking Penguin, New York

Fischer EP (2008) Das große Buch der Evolution. Fackelträger Verlag, Köln

Ganten D, Spahl T, Deichmann T (2009) Die Steinzeit steckt uns in den Knochen. Piper Verlag, München

Gluckman P, Beedle A, Hanson M (2009) Principles of evolutionary medicine. Oxford University Press, Oxford

Jahn I (2000) Geschichte der Biologie. Spektrum Akademischer Verlag GmbH, Heidelberg

Laberge AM, Michaud J, Richter A, Lemyre E, Lambert M, Brais B, Mitchell GA (2005) Population history and its impact on medical genetics in Quebec. Clin Genet 68:287–301

Mayr E (1982) The Growth of Biological Thought. The Belknap Press of Harvard University Press, Cambridge (Massachusetts)

Spalding KL, Arner E, Westermark PO, Bernard S, Buchholz BA, Bergmann O, Blomqvist L, Hoffstedt J, Naslund E, Britton T, Concha H, Hassan M, Ryden M, Frisen J, Arner P (2008) Dynamics of fat cell turnover in humans. Nature 453:783–787

Brain and Immune System—Two Competing Realms

Contents

3.1 **Energy Release—Competing Role of Brain and Immune System – 52**

3.2 **Energy Release—Mutual Immediate Assistance – 54**

3.3 **Energy Storage—Memory Function of Brain and Immune System – 55**
3.3.1 Brain's Memory – 56
3.3.2 Immune System Memory—Tetanus and So On – 56
3.3.3 Foreign Antigen, Autoantigen and Memory – 58

References – 60

3

It is like the unequal half-brothers Castor and Pollux, who were born on the same day and were inseparable. They were the patrons of Sparta, saviors in battles on land and at sea. Castor was a skilled horse tamer and Pollux a great boxer. Both took part in the voyages of Jason and the Argonauts, and they accompanied Hercules on his journey to the Amazons. They struggled hard, and the mortal Castor fell in battle. The immortal Pollux wanted to follow him into the realm of shadows, but Zeus forbade it, but granted daily alternating meetings of the two in the realm of Olympus and in the realm of shadows.

So inseparable are also the brain and the immune system. They guard the same body, each in its own realm, they meet daily and fight for the cause of the whole.

3.1 Energy Release—Competing Role of Brain and Immune System

In ▶ Chap. 1 and 2 the dominant role of the brain (and thus also of muscles, heart muscle, psychomotor unit) and the immune system in the respective acute context of a dangerous situation was highlighted. Now the separate and acute procurement measures must be examined more closely. The explanations are supported by ◘ Fig. 3.1, which is repeatedly referred to. Let the text guide you and always go to ◘ Fig. 3.1 to classify what you have learned.

In fight and flight, the brain activates the pituitary gland, the adrenal glands, and the sympathetic nervous system. These are the directly dependent control elements. The following hormones are released in this way during acute fight and flight:

- Cortisol,
- Adrenaline,
- Noradrenaline,
- Growth hormone,
- Thyroid hormones and
- the RAA hormones (according to ◘ Table 1.3).

These hormones all inhibit the effect of insulin on the three most important storage organs liver, adipose tissue, and muscles (not on the heart muscle). Remember: Insulin was the most important storage hormone. Energy-rich substrates are no longer stored and thus freely available in the bloodstream, showing that in this case the CAEN is essentially controlled by the selfish brain. This process is accompanied by acute loss of appetite (anorexia), and gastrointestinal activity is largely stopped. Or could you imagine eating and digesting a cream cake while fighting or fleeing? Take a quiet look at the upper half and the left side of ◘ Fig. 3.1 (arrow on "Inhibition of insulin action").

In the case of inflammation, on the other hand, it looks like this: Although an inflammatory reaction should be as local and limited as possible, inflammation can also involve the entire body. This is the case when cytokines or immune messengers enter the bloodstream and thus influence other organs, or when activated immune cells migrate in the bloodstream and find entry and influence in endocrine glands. A remote effect of cytokines is also possible via the activation of pain pathways,

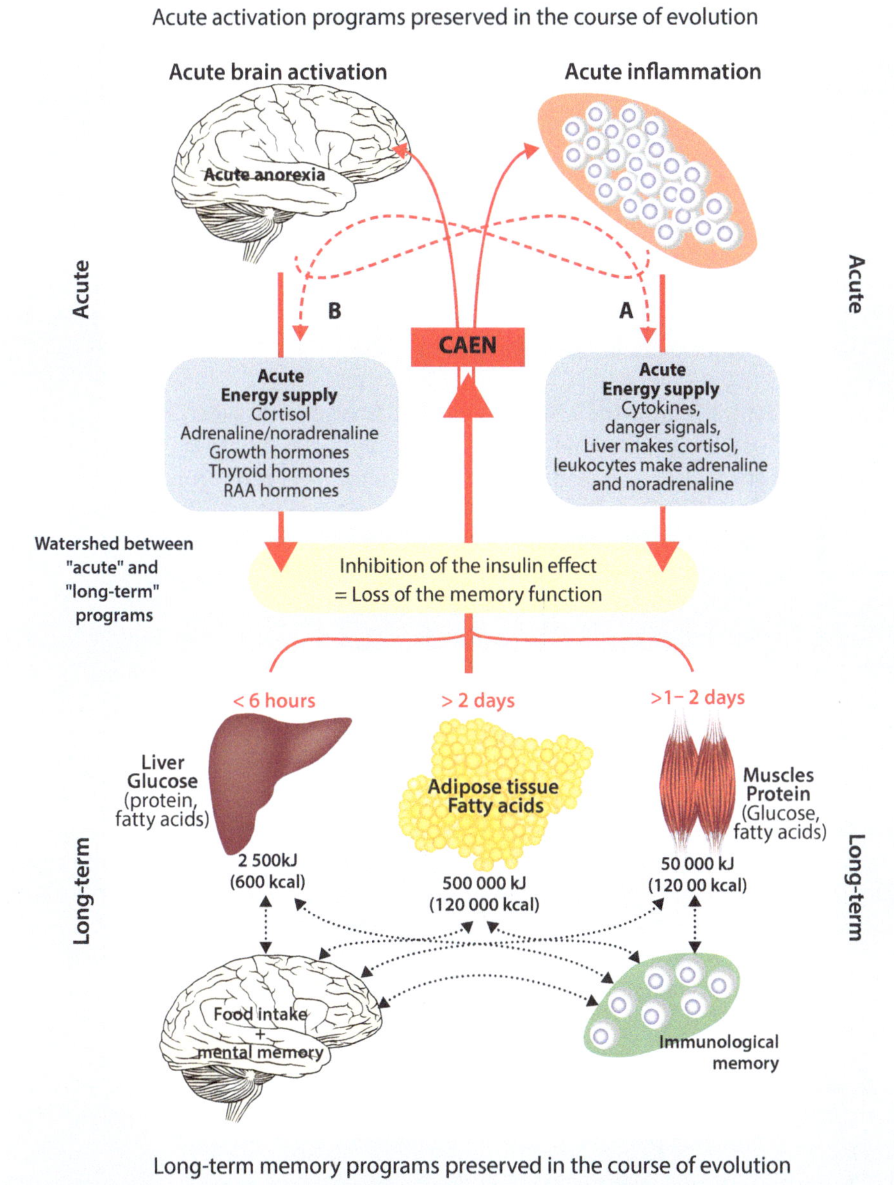

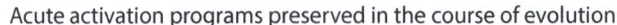

Acute activation programs preserved in the course of evolution

Acute brain activation

Acute inflammation

Acute anorexia

Acute

B

CAEN

A

Acute

**Acute
Energy supply**
Cortisol
Adrenaline/noradrenaline
Growth hormones
Thyroid hormones
RAA hormones

**Acute
Energy supply**
Cytokines,
danger signals,
Liver makes cortisol,
leukocytes make adrenaline
and noradrenaline

Watershed between
"acute" and
"long-term"
programs

Inhibition of the insulin effect
= Loss of the memory function

< 6 hours

> 2 days

>1– 2 days

Liver
Glucose
(protein,
fatty acids)

**Adipose tissue
Fatty acids**

Muscles
Protein
(Glucose,
fatty acids)

Long-term

2 500kJ
(600 kcal)

500 000 kJ
(120 000 kcal)

50 000 kJ
(120 00 kcal)

Long-term

Food intake
+
mental memory

Immunological
memory

Long-term memory programs preserved in the course of evolution

The two parts of acute energy provision (top) in contrast to the long-term program of energy storage (bottom).
This diagram is a central illustration in the book. The illustration should be clear from the text of this chapter, as
reference to this illustration is made repeatedly in the text.
The dashed arrows in the lower half show cross-connections to protect the energy stores. The thin arrows in the
upper half, labeled A and B, show the mutual immediate assistance of the two selfish realms. Further explanations
in the text.

■ **Fig. 3.1**   The two realms of acute energy provision (upper half) in contrast to the long-term program
of energy storage (lower half)

3

as cytokines trigger pain stimuli that can then be forwarded to the brain. For example, there is this involvement of the entire body in wound healing when the wound problem is large enough. Remember the man from New Guinea with the scratch wound who received antibiotics from the randomly arriving research traveler. In the case of the flu, there is a severe general inflammatory activity from the outset, which is accompanied by high blood levels of cytokines and many activated immune cells.

In contrast to the brain, the immune system uses
- the cytokines, the danger signals from dead cells,
- the activated and circulating immune cells and
- the independent production of hormones such as adrenaline , noradrenaline, growth hormone etc. in involved immune cells.

All these factors inhibit the effect of insulin. Energy-rich substrates are no longer stored and are freely available in the bloodstream. In this case, the CAEN is essentially controlled by the selfish immune system. This process is accompanied by acute loss of appetite (anorexia), and gastrointestinal activity is largely suspended.

The question may also be asked here whether one can eat and digest cream cake during a severe flu. Consider the top half and the right side of ◘ Fig. 3.1 (arrow pointing to "Inhibition of insulin action").

It is also telling that the factors of the respective dominant organ inhibit the other selfish system. Thus, cortisol, adrenaline, and noradrenaline can inhibit many important pro-inflammatory functions of the immune system. So when the selfish brain becomes active, it inhibits the immune system. Conversely, inflammation—more precisely cytokines and activated migrating immune cells—can slow down the brain and stress axes, which we perceive as fatigue, lethargy, increased need for sleep, and depressive symptoms during an infectious disease (*Sickness behavior*). So when the selfish immune system becomes active, it inhibits the brain and the stress axis hormones. This mutual inhibition becomes particularly necessary during prolonged activation of one or the other selfish system.

In the very acute phase—that is, within a few hours to a few days—there can also be mutual immediate assistance.

3.2 Energy Release—Mutual Immediate Assistance

In the upper part of ◘ Fig. 3.1, two thin arrows marked with (A) and (B) indicate a mutual activation of the brain on the one hand and the immune system on the other. So, are the brain and immune system not entirely independent of each other after all?

An activation of the brain indeed leads to a mild activation of the largely inactive immune system. The activation of the immune system during psychologically stressful events is evidenced by a two- to three-fold increase in the blood levels of interleukin-6. This then means an increase from about 1–2 pg/ml (picograms per milliliter) to 5 pg/ml. Is that a lot? No, it is not much, because in a proper inflammatory disease, interleukin-6 is increased to 100 pg/ml to 10,000 pg/ml. This merely gentle cross-activation may thus be an acute mild support reaction, but the brain is dominant with the hormones of the pituitary gland, the adrenal glands, and the sympathetic nervous system (i.e., the two stress axes).

Conversely, an activation of the immune system can be accompanied by an immediate activation of the brain if the immune response is large enough and affects the whole body. Thus, the pituitary gland, the adrenal glands, and the sympathetic nervous system can initially be stimulated. However, this activation does not last long, as a soon normalization of the two stress axes is observed. Studies in humans have shown that the injection of interleukin-6 or other cytokines does indeed cause a significant reaction in the short term, but long-term administration over a few days is hardly significant. After a few days of the most severe infection, a mild activation of the stress axes is still observed, so that the blood levels of cortisol and adrenaline are only slightly increased. This gentle cross-activation may thus be a mild support reaction, but the immune system is dominant with its independent possibilities of energy release, especially via the cytokines.

So, when we consider the two dominant realms of the brain and the immune system, the activated factors largely act independently of each other. Despite mutual immediate assistance from the respective other organ in short-term situations, one can therefore assume an egoistic, energy-demanding attitude of the two dominant realms.

However, it is noticeable that the activation of the two realms leads to a large shutdown of food intake (anorexia) and gastrointestinal activity. This shutdown has three serious implications:

- The organs in the liver-stomach-intestine area require a lot of energy, and the shutdown saves this energy.
- The organs in the liver-stomach-intestine area lose weight quickly when starved or when energy intake is stopped. Muscles lose less weight than abdominal organs.
- The short-term shutdown of gastrointestinal activity leads to complete dependence on reserves.

The latter fact is of extraordinary importance, as the supply of external energy-rich substrates (glucose, protein, fat), calcium, phosphate, magnesium, vitamins, and trace elements (e.g., iron) is thus prevented. In the context of these acute reactions (fight/flight and inflammation), energy reserves and existing stores of calcium, phosphate, magnesium, vitamins, and trace elements must therefore be accessed. It is therefore not surprising at all that both the factors of the stress axes (cortisol, noradrenaline, adrenaline, thyroid hormones, and the RAA hormones), but also the cytokines and immune cells directly break down the bone.

Let's now turn to the lower half of ▪ Fig. 3.1, which revisits energy storage (see also ▪ Fig. 1.8).

3.3 Energy Storage—Memory Function of Brain and Immune System

During normal life, programs of the brain and the immune system are also needed for long-term planning. After all, not everything is about fight, flight, and acute inflammation. There is also growth, repair, and reproduction, which require energy.

3

Under normal circumstances, without these acute survival programs and without the use of the associated energy provision factors, we lead a peaceful and healthy life. If we consume excess energy-rich substrates, we store them in the adipose tissue. The eating programs and satiety programs should serve a balanced food intake, with physical activity and thus muscle activity not being neglected, as otherwise the muscles shrink.

The brain has the ability to store important content, so that among other things, food-seeking behavior is stored.

3.3.1 Brain's Memory

It has been proven that humans and animals can particularly well remember those places that are rich in good food sources. This characteristic is very important for hunters and gatherers. For us modern humans, the knowledge of the location of supermarkets and wine shops is less important, although it is striking how everyone knows exactly where to get their favorite foods and drinks. Thus, food intake, food-seeking behavior, and storage for long-term use have been conserved throughout evolutionary history (◘ Fig. 3.1, lower half).

On the side of the immune system too, there are important programs that have nothing to do with acute inflammation and are needed in the long term. It is fascinating that both the brain and the immune system possess a **memory function**. There are no other organs with such a large memory function as the brain and the immune system (in a later book of 2020, I reported on the memory of fatty acids not mentioned here). This also speaks for the essential importance of the two selfish realms. Because if someone remembers something, it certainly has something to do with energy saving for hard times. We want to draw on an example from the energy industry for this.

If we store gas in a gas tank or crude oil in oil tanks, we do this because we want to keep energy available for scarce times. More than 40 years ago, in 1973, the OPEC countries turned off the oil tap to draw attention to the problems of the Arab-Israeli Yom Kippur War. There was an acute oil shortage with car-free Sundays because oil was scarce. The following year, the Federal Republic of Germany had to pay 17 billion Deutsch Marks more than the year before, and this had social and economic consequences. The Energy Security Act of November 1973 legally regulated the security of energy supply. However, gas tanks in a bell-shaped form were introduced in Germany as early as the 1930s.

And it is also an achievement of mental memory that someone remembers the gas tanks in times of crisis and knows how to turn the tap on. But what does the memory of the immune system look like?

3.3.2 Immune System Memory—Tetanus and So On

The immune system stores encounters with infectious agents in immunological memory. Each of us knows the importance of immunological memory. For example, when one gets a tetanus vaccination, the dangerous tetanus toxin is injected in minute amounts. The tetanus toxin is normally produced by tetanus bacteria in large quantities in case of illness, and this is dangerous because the tetanus toxin paralyzes nerve and thus muscle functions. However, if one only gets small amounts of the tetanus toxin, there is no lockjaw.

On the contrary: Now the immune system recognizes the foreign tetanus toxin and can react. This foreign protein, i.e. the tetanus toxin, is also called a foreign antigen. The immune system now develops a defense strategy by producing so-called antibodies that neutralize the tetanus toxin. The success of the vaccination can then also be measured by the number of antibodies against tetanus toxin in the blood; the more, the better. In ◘ Fig. 3.2a, the tetanus toxin is shown in spatial structure.

The effect of this tetanus vaccination lasts 10 years, which means 10 years of protection against tetanus. Then one must repeat the vaccination to be protected again for 10 years.

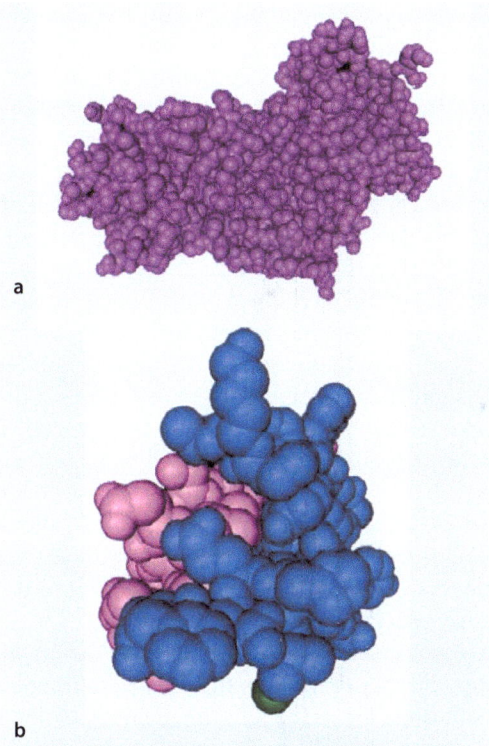

a

b

Spatial structure of tetanus toxin (top, foreign antigen) and insulin (bottom, autoantigen). The blue and pink spheres represent the amino acids in the molecule. Both are so small that they cannot be seen under a light microscope. These are models of the spatial arrangement of these two protein molecules. Tetanus toxin is a foreign antigen, whereas insulin is an autoantigen. These protein molecules are recognized by the antennae of the immune cells.

◘ **Fig. 3.2**   a, b Spatial structure of tetanus toxin (**a** foreign antigen) and insulin (**b** autoantigen)

Since the antibodies continue to be produced, there must be something like a memory of the immune system. If the tetanus toxin appears in our body during the 10 years, then the memory is activated, antibodies are produced against the foreign antigen, and the tetanus toxin is neutralized.

Great thing, such a vaccination, which by the way was carried out for the first time on a large scale in Constantinople in 1717 against smallpox on the orders of Sultan Ahmed III (1673–1736). The Englishman Edward Jenner then introduced a modified method in Bristol in 1796. He called it vaccination, because he got the vaccine material from cows with cowpox (vacca, lat. cow).

If we consider this memory in connection with tetanus, then we recognize here the confrontation with a foreign protein or foreign antigen. We also recognize an immunological memory against the foreign antigen. The immune system thus carries out an attack against foreign antigens. This attack has special characteristics that make us aware of the importance for energy saving.

At the first meeting of the immune cells and the foreign antigen, for example during a vaccination in early childhood, the immune system needs about 14 days until it can recognize and attack the foreign antigen at its best. It goes through a laborious maturation process, which takes place in the lymph nodes, the spleen, and the bone marrow. During this time, cell turnover is significantly increased (many cells are generated). These 14 days can really be long, as one experiences a significant feeling of illness during this time and also for a week afterwards. Remember the shutdown of food intake and the wasting time; the reserves are needed.

At the second meeting of the immune cells and the foreign antigen, for example during vaccination in advanced childhood (with the same vaccine), i.e. after the first meeting has taken place, the immune system now reacts much faster, as the memory function is switched on. Now there are already perfect immune cells from the start that immediately recognize the foreign antigen. Within 3–5 days, one already has a perfect immune response that neutralizes the foreign antigen. Thus, the tetanus bacteria can produce tetanus toxin, but the neutralizing response is available faster, and there is no lockjaw.

Compared to the 14 days at first contact, the effort of the immune system at second contact is much lower in terms of energy. In addition, we do not experience a severe feeling of illness at second contact and can eat and drink more or less normally. Here one clearly sees the energetic advantage.

This memory is often established in young years, which is why we do not have to go through many childhood diseases in older age. Imagine if we had chickenpox every 3 years. In terms of reinfection, the memory of the immune system plays a long-term energy-saving role (◘ Fig. 3.1, lower half). This long-term role was retained in evolutionary history in the context of infectious diseases against foreign antigens.

3.3.3 Foreign Antigen, Autoantigen and Memory

Now we were talking about a foreign antigen like tetanus toxin, which must be recognized and neutralized by the immune system. But what about the many protein molecules in our own body that could also be recognized as an antigen? These own antigens are called autoantigens as opposed to foreign antigens (autós, gr. self, own). Insulin, for example, is an autoantigen. Insulin, the storage hormone, consists of 51 individual amino acids strung together to form a protein clump (◘ Fig. 3.2b). Such protein clumps like insulin can be autoantigens, and these autoantigens can trigger an immune response, which is then called an autoimmune response. Many people show an autoimmune response to insulin, but it is usually completely harmless.

Unlike foreign antigens, harmless autoantigens lack the corresponding control signals for a full attack. This is similar to when the trumpeter sounds the attack during a hunt, but the trumpet doesn't work. The full attack is omitted, but the immune system still remembers the autoantigen in the immunological memory. It remembers there that the autoantigen must be "harmless" because it was not linked with a proper attack signal. The immunological memory recognizes the autoantigens and assigns them the meaning "own" and "harmless".

However, it can also happen that an autoantigen is presented in the context of foreign attack signals, such as during a viral or bacterial disease. Under such unfortunate circumstances, it can happen that the autoantigen is recognized as a foreign antigen and the attack is carried out in full force.

Here, the immune system makes a serious mistake, leading to a so-called autoimmune disease, a disease that is directed against the self. About 6% of the population suffer from autoimmune diseases. Where 94% of people benefit from the functions of the immune system in dealing with a foreign antigen, the same immune system leads to an autoimmune disease, a chronic inflammatory disease (examples: rheumatoid arthritis, thyroiditis, multiple sclerosis, psoriasis, lupus etc.) in 6%.

We want to end this section with a positive memory. The mental memory in the brain and the immunological memory serve to **save energy**. These two memory performances have been selected in the course of evolution because they are beneficial for the entire system. These elements play a central role in energy storage in ◘ Fig. 3.1 in the lower half.

In a nutshell

- The selfish brain activates the pituitary gland, the adrenal glands, and the sympathetic nervous system for energy procurement.
- In this way, hormones or neurotransmitters of the sympathetic nervous system are released during acute fight and flight, but also during psychological stress, which inhibit insulin (the storage hormone par excellence) or the insulin effect:
  - Cortisol,
  - Adrenaline,
  - Noradrenaline,
  - Growth hormone,
  - Thyroid hormone, and
  - the RAA hormones.
- The selfish immune system uses cytokines, danger signals, and migrating immune cells with their accompanying immune messengers for energy procurement.
- In this way, immune messengers are released during immune reactions that inhibit insulin or the insulin effect:
  - TNF,
  - Interleukin-6,
  - Danger signals,

3

- – Hormones from immune cells (noradrenaline),
- – Hormones from the liver (inflammation-induced stimulated cortisol).
- ▬ In longer-lasting situations, the factors of the selfish brain inhibit the selfish immune system and vice versa. In short-term situations, both help each other in a mild way (mutual immediate assistance).
- ▬ Loss of appetite accompanies the brain's fight and flight reaction, as well as the immune system's defense reaction. Therefore, the body must rely on stored energy-rich substrates, calcium, phosphate, magnesium, vitamins, and trace elements (e.g., iron) in these situations.
- ▬ The selfish brain and the selfish immune system each have their own memory, which serves to save energy. Only these two selfish organs have a memory (in a later publication of 2020, the author recognized a third memory: the memory of the fatty acid system).
- ▬ A foreign antigen is a molecule (usually a protein molecule) not belonging to our body, which is recognized by the immune system and bound and neutralized by antibodies.
  - – There is an immunological memory for "foreign".
  - – Example: Tetanus toxin.
- ▬ An autoantigen is a molecule (usually a protein molecule) belonging to our body, which is recognized by the immune system as "self" and "harmless".
  - – There is an immunological memory for "self".
  - – Example: Insulin.
- ▬ In an autoimmune disease, there is mistakenly an attack against a harmless, self-antigen. About 6% of people suffer from an autoimmune disease. In contrast, 94% of people benefit from the abilities of the immune system during infection.
- ▬ Between the acute activation phases of the selfish brain and the selfish immune system, there are peaceful intermediate phases that are used for growth, repair, and reproduction. To ensure these functions, the egoists—the brain and the immune system—must be largely tamed.

References

Dorn LD, Susman EJ, Pabst S, Huang B, Kalkwarf H, Grimes S (2008) Association of depressive symptoms and anxiety with bone mass and density in ever-smoking and never-smoking adolescent girls. Arch Pediatr Adolesc Med 162:1181–1188

Ramsey JJ, Harper ME, Weindruch R (2000) Restriction of energy intake, energy expenditure, and aging. Free Radic Biol Med 29:946–968

Straub RH (2020). The memory of the fatty acid system. Prog Lipid Res. 79:101049. doi: ▶ https://doi.org/10.1016/j.plipres.2020.101049

Wahlbeck K, Forsen T, Osmond C, Barker DJ, Eriksson JG (2001) Association of schizophrenia with low maternal body mass index, small size at birth, and thinness during childhood. Arch Gen Psychiatry 58:48–52

Energy Expenditure in the Spotlight

The immune system, which we exposed as selfish in the first part, creates many problems throughout the body when there is an inflammation that is prolonged and severe. The author of the book has gathered much experience in the field of chronic rheumatic diseases, especially rheumatoid arthritis, polymyalgia rheumatica, and chronic inflammatory bowel diseases. Historically, the focus of the observations was initially on the rather "severe inflammations". These severe inflammations can obscure the view of the "milder inflammatory states". Moreover, in these severe inflammatory diseases, the immune system is very selfish, which becomes particularly visible when the diseases are not yet or not well treated. The energy expenditure by the immune system can then be quite enormous.

During the course of scientific work, it became clear that even milder forms of inflammation, coupled with additional energy-consuming processes, for example during aging, can create very similar long-term problems as observed in rheumatic diseases. Unlike rheumatic diseases, which can quickly cause high inflammatory activity and energy expenditure, the processes during aging are more protracted and cumulative. Several energy-consuming factors from different areas come together, but lead to similar problems.

In Part II of the book, the various conditions that can lead to more energy expenditure are examined in more detail. This is an important platform to better assess the situation, especially when it comes to aging.

In Part III of the book, we then discuss the long-term problems of increased energy expenditure. You will recognize that the problems addressed can be explained with the help of the energy considerations and evolutionary medicine from Part I and Part II.

Inflammation and Energy

Contents

4.1   Historical Definition of Inflammation – 64

4.2   Inflammation Strength: Rose Thorn, Rheumatism, and Sepsis – 65

4.3   Inflammation Causes Increased Energy Expenditure – 67

References – 72

4.1 Historical Definition of Inflammation

Historically, inflammation has been described since Celsus (writer in Rome; around 25 BCE to about 50 ACE) and Galen (physician in Rome; 129 to 210 ACE) with the five cardinal symptoms (see Infobox).

The Five Cardinal Symptoms of Inflammation
- 1) Redness
- 2) Heat
- 3) Swelling
- 4) Pain
- 5) Loss of function

All points are recognizable in ▪ Fig. 4.1, with points 1–4 becoming visible primarily in the lower image (▪ Fig. 4.1b) (arrow). The clinical picture of the hands (above, ▪ Fig. 4.1a) makes it clear that this must inevitably result in functional restrictions. A surgical image showing the cartilage layer would make it clear that there is inflamed tissue that replaces the normal cartilage tissue. It looks as if a red weed is growing over the healthy yellowish cartilage layer, as described in H.G. Wells' *War of the Worlds*, where the red weed from Mars overgrows the Earth. The healthy tissue is replaced by a red—well-perfused—inflamed tissue.

Inflamed tissue means that immune cells migrate and local cells are activated. Furthermore, there is a dilation of blood vessels.

- The redness is best explained by the larger number of red blood cells per area in the context of inflammatory vasodilation.
- The heat is explained by the fact that the vessels are wide open and warmer blood enters the inflammation region.
- The swelling occurs because vessels become leaky. This leakiness is important in a wound event because it allows migrating immune cells to enter the inflammation area in the first place.
- If we see something like this in a chronic inflammatory disease, then we must realize that this mechanism was retained in connection with acute wound infections in our evolutionary history (not for the chronic inflammatory disease).
- Pain arises because inflammation factors activate the pain nerve fibers. The explanations on the topic of pain will be taken up again in more detail in the next chapter (▶ Chap. 5).

If inflammation exists only for a short period of time, it is usually a positive sign that contributes to the elimination of an infectious agent, the cleaning of a wound, the removal of a foreign body, and wound repair. We found in ▶ Chap. 2 "Evolutionary Medicine" that inflammation cannot persist for long because of a possible high energy consumption. We also learned that the immune system is selfish and therefore cannot claim high energy resources for itself in the long term. If inflammation becomes protracted, subsequent problems arise, which we will deal with in the third part of the book.

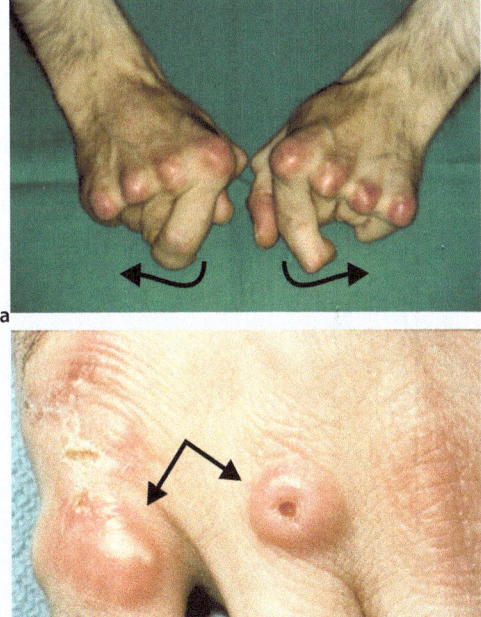

Typical changes in the severe joint inflammation
known as rheumatoid arthritis.
a) Change in the joint position.
b) Redness and swelling as well as nodules along the
extensor tendons of muscles that move the fingers
(rheumatoid nodules)

◘ **Fig. 4.1**   a, b Typical changes in severe joint inflammation named rheumatoid arthritis. **a** Joint deformation. **b** Redness and swelling as well as nodules along the extensor tendons of muscles that move the
fingers (rheumatoid nodules)

Before that, we want to take a closer look at the strength of the inflammation
and the energy consumption of inflammation.

4.2 Inflammation Strength: Rose Thorn, Rheumatism, and Sepsis

Imagine an armed confrontation where the opposing parties each use a pistol
with one shot of ammunition, e.g., as in Thomas Mann's famous novel *The Magic
Mountain*, when Lodovico Settembrini meets Leo Naphta. The pistol shot reaches
about 100 meters and has a small harmless energy of less than 0.5 kJ at the point of
impact. This pistol fight therefore has only a low strength and spread. After all, it
costs little energy.

On the other hand, a 1200 kg explosive shell from the "Big Bertha" of the First
World War flies about 9 kilometers and has an impact energy of 58,000 kJ. This is

by no means harmless, especially since the explosive shell explodes on impact, releasing even more devastating energy, a total of 1 million kJ. If you compare the explosive shell of the Big Bertha with the atomic bomb *Fat Man*, which exploded over Nagasaki in the Second World War, the energy of the explosive shell in relative units is slightly larger than that of a bullet in relation to the explosive shell of the Big Bertha. The atomic bomb of Nagasaki had a released energy of about 84 billion kJ.

If you translate this into the warlike events during an immune system's inflammatory reaction, the bullet can be compared to a rose thorn that has penetrated the skin, but the atomic bomb can be compared to a severe sepsis. In one case, we have a locally limited immune reaction, in which fewer local immune cells and local energy reserves are involved, and which does not spread. In the other case, the entire body is affected, a countless number of immune cells are in use, and large energy reserves are needed. The daily consumption can increase from 10,000 kJ (2388 kcal) to 15,000 kJ (4777 kcal) in the case of sepsis. Here, the strength is high, and the area of spread is equivalent to the entire body.

The erythrocyte sedimentation rate, the blood levels of C-reactive protein or Interleukin-6 have proven to be very good measures for the strength of inflammation in the human body. If the general practitioner wants to rule out inflammation, he uses at least one of these parameters. All three factors are closely related, with the cytokine Interleukin-6 being very important because it stimulates the other two factors from the liver. Since it is at the beginning of the cause-effect chain, Interleukin-6—the hormone of inflammation—is significant.

A young person at the age of 20 has an Interleukin-6 level of 1 pg/ml, which increases to about 2.5 pg/ml as they age until 70 years. This shows the increase of a mild inflammatory constellation during aging. If an old, but otherwise healthy person is placed in a new home, for example in a nursing home, this psychological stress combined with age already leads to an increase of Interleukin-6 to 3.5 pg/ml. In life events associated with increased stress, such as the long-term care of a relative with Alzheimer's, Interleukin-6 increases to about 6 pg/ml.

A well-adjusted rheumatic or autoimmune disease shows Interleukin-6 levels of about 8–10 pg/ml, and this should always be the goal of the treating physician. He may possibly follow the erythrocyte sedimentation rate or the C-reactive protein, but these should preferably be near the upper normal value or even below it. In one of our studies on rheumatoid arthritis at the University Hospital Regensburg, the levels of Interleukin-6 before therapy were 26.0 pg/ml and after successful therapy 8.5 pg/ml. In another study on patients with rheumatoid arthritis, the Interleukin-6 level decreased within the first week of therapy from 65.3 pg/ml to 14.1 pg/ml. Here, the doctor knows that the therapy was good, as the inflammation decreased significantly in a very short time and will continue to decrease. The faster the inflammation values decrease, the more favorable is the prognosis regarding joint damage.

In another study on patients with sepsis, conducted at the University Hospital in Regensburg, patients had an average of 2910 pg/ml Interleukin-6 in the first week after hospital admission, 359 pg/ml in the second week, and 211 pg/ml in the third week. So, it got better over time. In this study, one patient's Interleukin-6 level was determined to be 107,259 pg/ml. This is the atomic bomb of inflammation.

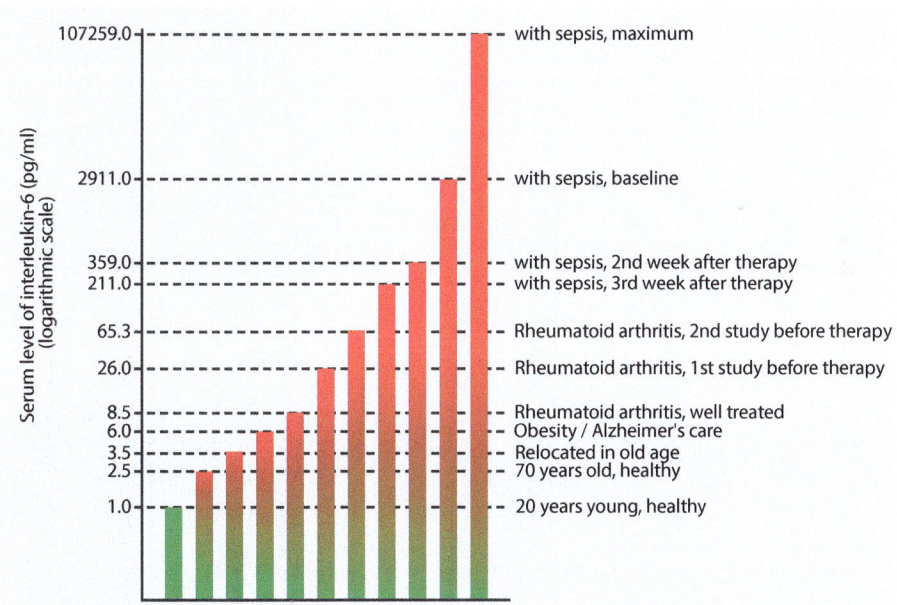 Figure 4.2 summarizes these findings graphically. It becomes clear there that the inflammation—measured by the level of Interleukin-6—can vary in strength from 1.0 pg/ml to 100,000 pg/ml. Obviously, 1 pg/ml corresponds to a situation without inflammation, whereas 1000–100,000 pg/ml represent a strong inflammation. However, it is not easy to draw the exact line between "weak" and "strong", as people are very different in their sensitivity. Moreover, one can probably only guess the full extent of the situation with a single factor like Interleukin-6.

4.3 Inflammation Causes Increased Energy Expenditure

In a frequently cited study of healthy individuals, a working group at the American National Institute of Health in Washington demonstrated that the administration of Interleukin-6 via injection under the skin increased the levels of the same Interleukin-6 and that this led to an increased energy expenditure of the entire body (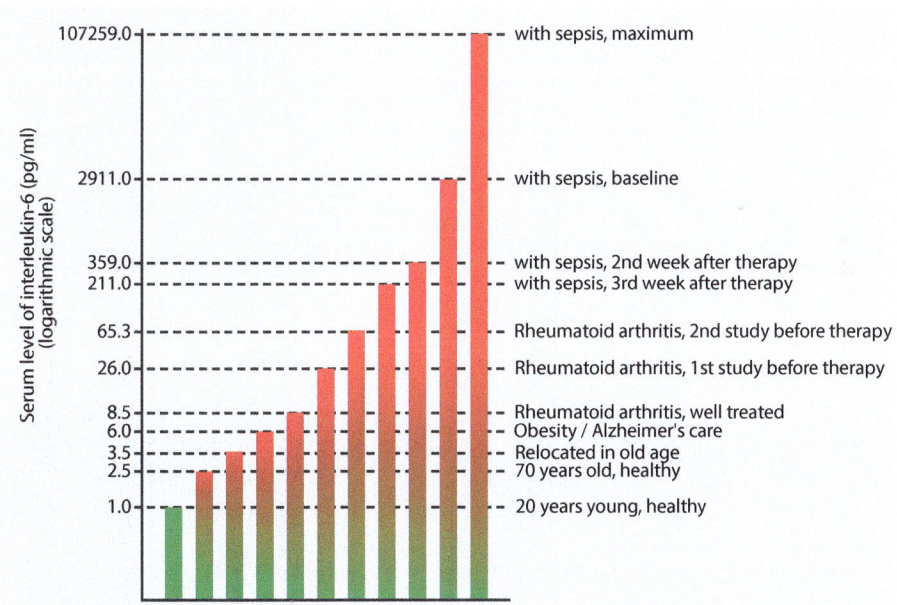 Fig. 4.3).

If the levels of Interleukin-6 were increased from the usual 1 pg/ml to 6 pg/ml, then the energy expenditure increased by 250 kJ (60 kcal) per day (Fig. 4.3). If

Serum level of interleukin-6 in different states. A logarithmic scale was used for the y-axis, which is often used for exponential growth. The green color indicates the normal situation. With higher inflammation, the color changes to red, indicating a more severe inflammatory situation. In rheumatoid arthritis, two examples are given for the serum value of interleukin-6 before the start of therapy, because this disease can begin more or less strongly (some patients have serum values of up to 200 pg/ml). The maximum in the sepsis study occurred in one patient. The other data on sepsis are mean values from a very large number of patients.
Obesity (= obesity) is defined as a body mass index (BMI) (= weight in kg divided by height in meters squared) of 30 kg/m² or more.

Fig. 4.2 Serum levels of Interleukin-6 in different states

4

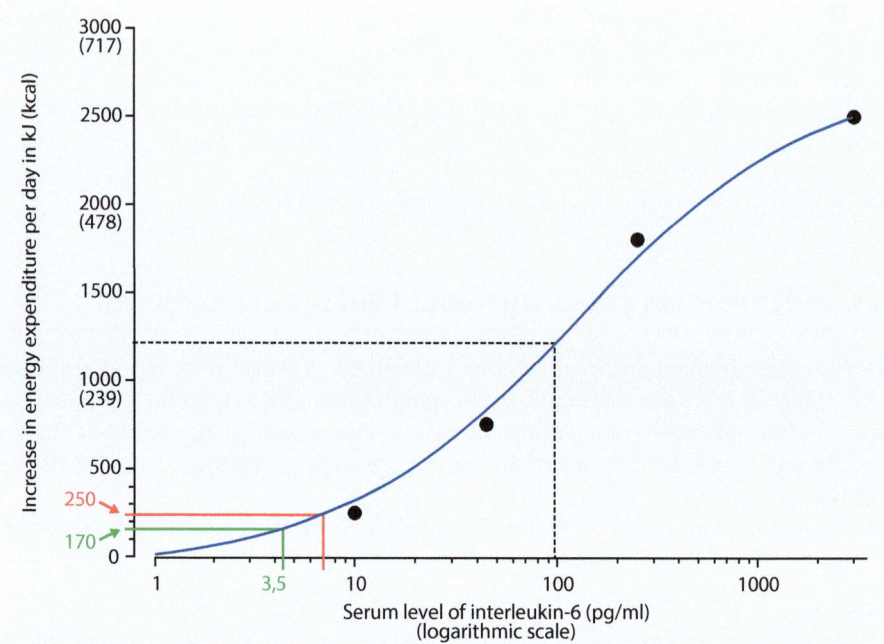

The rise in the interleukin-6 level increases energy expenditure per day. The cytokine interleukin-6 was injected under the skin of the test subjects using a syringe. After a short time, the blood level of interleukin-6 rose to the indicated values (black dots). At the same time, the increase in energy expenditure above the normal basal metabolic rate was measured. For example, 500 kJ on the Y-axis means a 500 kJ increase in energy expenditure due to the injection of interleukin-6 and the associated increase in inflammation. The blue curve has been determined in such a way that the black measuring points of the test subjects lie as precisely as possible on the curve. It can be seen that with increasing levels of the interleukin-6 on the X-axis, the energy expenditure on the Y-axis increases. If the blood level increases to 3.5 pg/ml (green lines), the energy expenditure increases by 170 kJ (40 kcal) per day. If the level is increased to 6.0 pg/ml (red lines), the energy expenditure increases accordingly to 250 kJ per day. If the level is increased to 100 pg/ml (black dashed lines), the energy expenditure increases by around 1200 kJ per day.

□ **Fig. 4.3**   Increase in Interleukin-6 levels increases energy expenditure per day

a patient with a rheumatic disease is well treated, then the level of Interleukin-6 is at 10 pg/ml. In the experiment on healthy individuals, the increase from the usual 1 pg/ml to 10 pg/ml led to an increase in energy expenditure by 300 kJ (72 kcal) per day.

Now, 250 kJ and 300 kJ are not a very large amount from an energy perspective, as these additional expenditures would shorten the emaciation time in a modern human in a sedentary way of life with complete food stop from 55 days to 53 days. It becomes clear that this additional energy expenditure is insignificant, and this is also evident when considering the energy expenditure in □ Table 1.1.

The situation is quite different with the high levels of Interleukin-6 of 1000–3000 pg/ml in □ Fig. 4.3, which lead to an increase in energy expenditure by 2500 kJ (600 kcal) per day. These additional expenditures would shorten the emaciation time with complete food stop in a modern human from 55 to 44 days. This is then similar to the example with the flu disease, which was used in the calculation of the emaciation time in ▪ Table 1.2. With such a shortening of the emaciation time by so many days, one must assume a strong inflammation. A pregnant woman needs about 474 kJ (113 kcal) more energy per day according to ▪ Table 1.1 and when breastfeeding about 1778 kJ (425 kcal). Both values should make it clear to us in relation to the 2500 kJ (600 kcal) mentioned in this section that a severe inflammation can hardly be reconciled with these other things.

In this example of the working group at the American National Institute of Health, only Interleukin-6 was injected, and this is known to be only one factor of inflammation. To better illuminate the relationship between several factors of inflammation and energy expenditure, instead of Interleukin-6, several factors would have to be injected simultaneously, and something similar has been done by a Swiss working group from Lausanne in humans.

The Swiss simulated a bacterial disease in humans by injecting bacterial components. These components cannot multiply, which is why the inflammation triggered by them is short-term and therefore largely harmless. From an ethical point of view, such studies can be carried out on small groups of normal individuals. In addition, only small amounts are administered, so that at most a moderate inflammatory situation is established for a short time (12 hours). Unlike with Interleukin-6, however, this procedure releases many factors of the immune cells, and this could significantly influence energy expenditure.

In fact, this approach resulted in significantly higher energy expenditure of 2100 kJ (500 kcal) per day, although the level of Interleukin-6 only rose to 100 pg/ml. If you look at ▪ Fig. 4.3, you can see that an increase in Interleukin-6 to 100 pg/ml would only result in an additional energy expenditure of about 1200 kJ (287 kcal). In the Swiss experiment, however, the energy expenditure is almost twice as high, and this can be explained as follows: With the injection of Interleukin-6, only the Interleukin-6 increases, and only this one inflammation factor then stimulates the energy expenditure. With the injection of bacterial components, however, in addition to Interleukin-6, the pro-inflammatory TNF also increases. In the Swiss experiments, TNF increased from 1.0 pg/ml to 150 pg/ml. Other factors of the immune system were not measured, but it can be assumed that there could be more such messenger substances of the immune cells measurable. It can be concluded that bacterial components cause a much broader immune response and thus higher energy expenditure.

The increased energy expenditures observed in the Swiss experiment can be considered significant. They would reduce the known emaciation time from 55 to 45 days. It is quite astonishing that a small amount of bacterial components stimulates such a strong energy expenditure. If an inflammatory rheumatic disease occurs for the first time, is not yet treated, and many inflammation factors (cytokines) are significantly increased, then we may have a similar constellation. There is a broad inflammatory response with a high energy expenditure.

In children with chronic arthritis and fresh joint inflammation, it was observed that energy expenditure was 21% higher compared to healthy, same-aged, and same-weight children. Extrapolated to the situation in adults, who consume about 10,000 kJ

4

(2388 kcal) per day, this would be 2100 kJ (500 kcal) more. This is very similar to the injection of bacterial components in the Swiss experiment. Other studies have clearly established the link between inflammation and increasing energy expenditure. Accordingly, energy expenditure increases by 15–25% when individuals suffer from a rheumatic disease.

At this point, we would like to briefly introduce another important factor of inflammation, the C-reactive protein (or CRP). Typically, our general practitioners measure the C-reactive protein or the erythrocyte sedimentation rate rather than interleukin-6 when they want to know something about inflammation. However, for all three one can say, the higher the value, the stronger the inflammation. It would therefore be interesting to know whether there is a similarly good correlation between the blood levels of C-reactive protein and the energy expenditure per day. This correlation in rheumatic patients was examined by us in collaboration with an Italian group from Marcon near Venice. ▪ Figure 4.4 shows the correlation in patients with rheumatoid arthritis.

At this point, it also becomes clear that in chronic inflammatory diseases, the inflammation must primarily be fought to get the energy expenditure and thus the subsequent problems under control. Nowadays, this can sometimes be done very specifically by neutralizing cytokines such as interleukin-6 and TNF directly. However, these therapies are very expensive, which is why highly effective but cheaper drugs with similar success are first administered in the therapeutic ladder. We will not discuss the therapies of these diseases further at this point, as this would go beyond the scope of the book.

Once again, we can summarize that inflammation consumes a lot of energy. This statement applies to the acute injection of interleukin-6 or bacterial components as well as to the onset of a chronic inflammatory disease. However, it could be that inflammation is not the sole cause of an increase in energy expenditure. Accompanying pain could also cause an increase in energy expenditure, and we will address this in the next chapter (▶ Chap. 5).

In a nutshell

- The historical definition of inflammation includes the important symptoms: redness, heat, swelling, pain, and loss of function (cardinal symptoms).
- We distinguish between weak, local inflammations (rose thorn, the gunshot) and strong, widespread inflammations (sepsis, the atomic bomb).
- Interleukin-6 is a good measure of the strength of inflammation. A boundary between "healthy" and "inflammatory" is at about 3–5 pg/ml interleukin-6 in the blood.
- During the aging process, the blood level of interleukin-6 slightly increases to 2–3 pg/ml.
- Acute inflammatory conditions such as after injection of interleukin-6 or bacterial components increase the energy expenditure of the entire body.
- The more factors (e.g., the cytokines interleukin-6 and TNF) are activated by the acute stimulus, the higher the energy expenditure. Comparing the injection of interleukin-6 alone with the injection of bacterial components, the latter generate significantly higher energy expenditure.

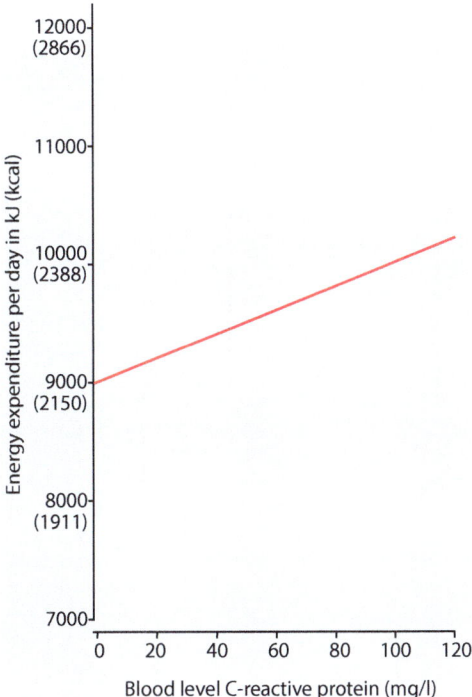

Relationship between blood levels of C-reactive protein and energy expenditure per day in patients with rheumatoid arthritis. Here, blood levels of C-reactive protein and energy expenditure per day were measured simultaneously in patients with rheumatoid arthritis. If there is no inflammation and the blood level of C-reactive protein is 0 mg/l, then the daily energy expenditure in this group of patients with different weights is around 9,000 kJ (2,150 kcal). This is where the red line intersects the y-axis. At very high values of C reactive protein on the right side of the x-axis, the values exceed 10,000 kJ (2,388 kcal) per day (right end of the red line). So you can see an increase of about 1,000 kJ (239 kcal) from the far left to the far right. The data comes from a scientific collaboration between the author and Dario Boschiero, Marcon, Italy.

◘ **Fig. 4.4** Correlation between the blood levels of C-reactive protein and the energy expenditure per day in patients with rheumatoid arthritis

- The C-reactive protein is another measure of inflammation that is associated with increased energy expenditure.
- Chronic inflammatory diseases such as chronic joint inflammation (arthritis) increase energy expenditure similarly to after injection of bacterial components.
- However, in these chronic inflammatory diseases, energy expenditure is constantly increased. Chronic autoimmune diseases are associated with high energy expenditure, especially when they are not well or not at all treated.

4

References

Knops N, Wulffraat N, Lodder S, Houwen R, de MK (1999) Resting energy expenditure and nutritional status in children with juvenile rheumatoid arthritis. J Rheumatol 26:2039–2043

Lutgendorf SK, Garand L, Buckwalter KC, Reimer TT, Hong SY, Lubaroff DM (1999) Life stress, mood disturbance, and elevated interleukin-6 in healthy older women. J Gerontol A Biol Sci Med Sci 54:M434–M439

Metsios GS, Stavropoulos-Kalinoglou A, Panoulas VF, Koutedakis Y, Nevill AM, Douglas KM, Kita M, Kitas GD (2008) New resting energy expenditure prediction equations for patients with rheumatoid arthritis. Rheumatology (Oxford) 47:500–556

Michaeli B, Martinez A, Revelly JP, Cayeux MC, Chiolero RL, Tappy L, Berger MM (2012) Effects of endotoxin on lactate metabolism in humans. Crit Care 16:R139

Straub RH, Georgi J, Helmke K, Vaith P, Lang B (2002) In polymyalgia rheumatica serum prolactin is positively correlated with the number of typical symptoms but not with typical inflammatory markers. Rheumatology (Oxford) 41:423–429

Straub RH, Müller-Ladner U, Lichtinger T, Schölmerich J, Menninger H, Lang B (1997) Decrease of interleukin 6 during the first 12 months is a prognostic marker for clinical outcome during 36 months treatment with disease-modifying anti-rheumatic drugs. Br J Rheumatol 36:1298–1303

Straub RH, Zeuner M, Lock G, Schölmerich J, Lang B (1997) High prolactin and low dehydroepiandrosterone sulphate serum levels in patients with severe systemic sclerosis. Br J Rheumatol 36:426–432

Tsigos C, Papanicolaou DA, Defensor R, Mitsiadis CS, Kyrou I, Chrousos GP (1997) Dose effects of recombinant human interleukin-6 on pituitary hormone secretion and energy expenditure. Neuroendocrinology 66:54–62

Pain and Energy

Contents

5.1   The Pain Receptors and Pain Stabilization – 74

5.2   Inflammation Causes Pain—The Sixth Sense – 75

5.3   When the Muscle Becomes Acidic, It Hurts – 76

5.4   Heat, Cold, and Pepper—Where Does It Reach the Brain? – 76

5.5   Acute and Chronic Pain – 77

5.6   Electric Shock, Pain, and Energy Expenditure – 78

5.7   Heat, Cold and Energy Expenditure – 79

        References – 80

© The Author(s), under exclusive license to Springer-Verlag GmbH, DE, part of Springer Nature 2024
R. H. Straub, *Understanding Aging, Fatigue, and Inflammation*,
https://doi.org/10.1007/978-3-662-68904-2_5

5.1 The Pain Receptors and Pain Stabilization

We experience pain in order to recognize injuries and functional disorders in the body and then to treat them. Acute pain warns us and leads to corresponding actions such as removing triggers, resting, seeking help, and ultimately healing. Pain was not abolished in the process of evolution but retained to learn avoidance strategies and initiate appropriate help actions quickly.

In our body, nerve fibers exist in almost all tissues, sending pain stimuli from the periphery to the central control areas in the spinal cord and brain. Pain can arise from mechanical stimuli, temperature stimuli, or chemical stimuli. In the various tissues, there are different receiver antennas for the different types of stimuli, let's call them pain receptors. Such a pain receptor can be found at the peripheral end of a pain nerve fiber. The other, central end of the pain nerve fiber is located in the spinal cord.

For the chemical and thermal stimuli, there is a very sophisticated pain receptor, which is shown in ◘ Fig. 5.1.

In the spinal cord, the inputs from the pain nerve fibers are controlled. If the pain stimulus is strong enough, then the signal is switched to long nerve pathways to the brain, and the pain signal finally reaches the cerebral cortex, where the pain enters consciousness and brings about a corresponding action and usually triggers negative feelings.

Interestingly, pain stimuli experience an extraordinary stabilization. Instead of stabilization, this is also called sensitization because the pain stimulus is amplified and one becomes more sensitive. A painful event must not simply be pushed aside,

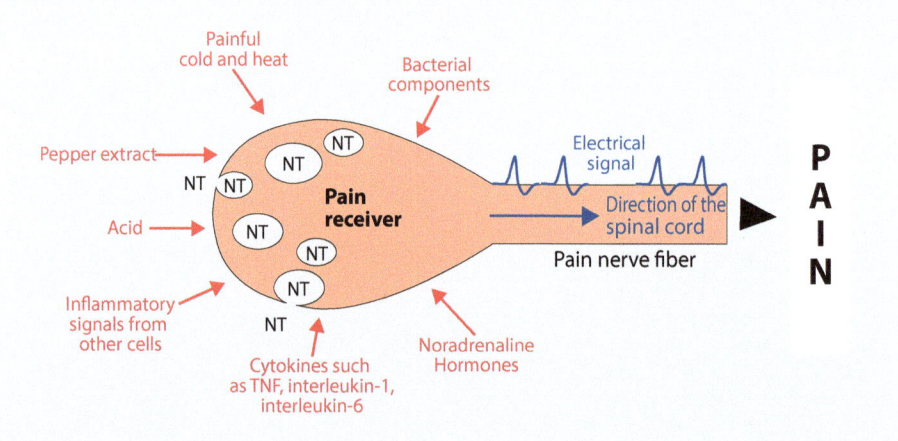

Pain receptor at the end of a pain nerve fiber. Various stimuli can sensitize the pain receptor so that an electrical signal is sent along the pain fibre to the spinal cord. If the pain receptor is stimulated strongly enough, it releases neurotransmitters (NT), which perform various functions around the nerve endings. The neurotransmitter "substance P" can, for example, activate local immune cell, attract defense cells and dilate the vessels in the surrounding area, causing redness, overheating of the area and the migration of immune cell (not shown in the picture).

◘ **Fig. 5.1**   Pain receptor at the end of a pain nerve fiber

as a helping action is immediately required. This sensitization occurs at various levels:

- at the pain receptor itself,
- on the pain nerve fibers,
- at the central switching point in the spinal cord, and
- very centrally in the brain.

However, the brain can also control the input of pain and partly contain it.

Acute pain can thus be inhibited by the body's own, morphine-like substances. Yes, we have our own poppy seeds, which produce morphine-like substances at various points in the body. Whether a pain is stabilized or contained depends on the strength of the pain stimulus. Strong stimuli must not be ignored, whereas light stimuli may also be suppressed. It also depends on our condition, as less stressed, rested, and endurance-trained people can better controll pain. Here, endurance sports take on a very important meaning.

5.2 Inflammation Causes Pain—The Sixth Sense

Inflammatory stimuli such as bacterial components, cytokines like TNF, Interleukin-1 and Interleukin-6, and various danger signals from immune cells and other body cells can directly activate the pain receptors (Fig. 5.1). In this respect, the state of inflammation can literally be measured and this information can be directly transmitted to the brain via the pain nerve fiber. Edwin Blalock from Birmingham, Alabama, once called this in a review article in the 1980s "the sixth sense," because it represents a kind of sensory perception in addition to the known five classical senses—seeing, hearing, smelling, tasting, and touching.

However, one should not imagine the measurement of this sensory impression as with a measuring device, so that we become aware of an exact extent of the inflammation. Since the sensation triggers many activations also below the level of consciousness, the whole thing is rather associated with a general feeling of illness and a local perception of pain.

In recent years, it has become increasingly clear that pain nerve fibers are responsible for this transmission of inflammation. This transmission of inflammatory states was discovered on the vagus nerve, which we got to know in the energy storage in Fig. 1.8. And as it sometimes happens in science, this important discovery was made simultaneously by two different groups in France and the USA in 1994. The two working groups subsequently argued about the priority.

In the following years, the same finding was also demonstrated for pain nerve fibers in the skin or in the throat. Think of throat pain after a night of heavy drinking, in which you smoked and consumed high-proof alcohol. An inflammation has spread in the throat, and cytokines are wreaking havoc in the local tissue. The inflammatory factors in the throat mucosa then activate the pain nerve fibers. Throat pain occurs.

Another working group from Jena (neurophysiology) has particularly dealt with the pain nerve fibers in joints. These pain nerve fibers can be activated by cytokines such as TNF, Interleukin-1 and Interleukin-6. Since joints are particularly well supplied with pain nerve fibers, the strength of inflammation in the joints should be particularly well measured and transmitted to the brain. And this is indeed the case, because inflamed joints are extremely painful.

5.3   When the Muscle Becomes Acidic, It Hurts

Others investigated pain in connection with oxygen deprivation in the tissue. Why is oxygen deprivation, for example in the case of a heart attack or vascular occlusion in the leg, so painful? We had already mentioned in the consideration of the energy-rich substrates (glucose, fatty acids and amino acids) in ▶ Chap. 1 "Energy and Body" that the energy-rich fuels are used in the presence of oxygen to produce the energy coin ATP (◘ Fig. 1.3). But when oxygen fails, as is the case with vascular occlusion, glucose is primarily used, as glucose can also be used to produce ATP in an oxygen-poor environment. Do you remember? However, this has a major disadvantage, because glucose in the tissue is directly broken down to lactate (lactic acid) and lactate is an acid.

When you exercise, the accumulation of lactate in the muscle can also become a problem because the oxygen supply is insufficient. If the removal of lactate via the veins is less than the new production from the muscle cells, then the muscle becomes acidic. This is then called: "The muscle becomes sore (german, sauer)" So if lactate is primarily produced in the case of oxygen deprivation, then this acid increasingly accumulates in the tissue.

Take another look at ◘ Fig. 5.1. On the left side of the pain receptor, the word "acid" is written. This very acid can activate the pain receptor, so that pain can occur with acidification with lactate (lactic acid), the breakdown product of glucose. In addition, in an oxygen-deprived tissue, the cytokines TNF, Interleukin-1 and Interleukin-6 are increasingly formed, which can also activate the pain receptor.

Oxygen deprivation is a strong inflammatory signal, so that very soon the pain receptor of ◘ Fig. 5.1 and then the centers in the spinal cord and brain are activated in various ways. That's why vascular occlusions quickly become very painful.

5.4   Heat, Cold, and Pepper—Where Does It Reach the Brain?

Another type of pain triggering occurs through painful heat and cold. Both can trigger a signal at the pain receptor that is transmitted from the periphery to the brain. It is now fascinating that the antenna for painful heat is simultaneously the antenna for acid and also for pepper extracts (◘ Fig. 5.1). Some people perceive pepper on the tongue as a pain stimulus. Thus, heat, acid, inflammation, and also pepper substances, which are produced in the body during inflammation and oxygen deficiency, are closely linked. The pain receptor integrates the various signals and sends a corresponding signal from the periphery to the spinal cord and into the brain when a threshold is exceeded. The pain penetrates into consciousness.

We want to summarize once again that many inflammation factors can cause excitation of the pain nerve fiber. In contrast to inflammation factors circulating in the blood, such as interleukin-6, the local activation of pain receptors and pain nerve fibers is very location-dependent. Many pain nerve fibers are located in the fingers, the hand, the toes, the foot, the lips, the face, the tongue, and in the throat. These are the most sensitive regions of the body, and these areas are particularly well represented in the brain (◘ Fig. 5.2). When inflammation is present in these regions, the inflammatory pain is particularly strong.

5.5 Acute and Chronic Pain

Acute pain usually lasts only a few days to a maximum of 2 weeks. They are associated with an acute activation of the body—e.g., the stress axes. We can quickly initiate the right actions here and control the pain very soon. The pain subsides soon, which is why we call it acute.

Chronic pain lasts weeks to months and even years. It is often associated with abnormal sensations (e.g., normal touch is felt as electrification), mental exhaustion, depression, and altered performance of all kinds. When chronic pain is present, the same acute stimuli are responsible at the beginning and possibly also in the further course, as we have learned in ◘ Fig. 5.1. In the case of tumor pain, inflammation pain, and pain due to oxygen deficiency, the known inflammatory factors such as cytokines, danger signals, and tissue acidosis are important factors. Compression of nerve fibers leads to continuous irritation of the pain nerve fibers and

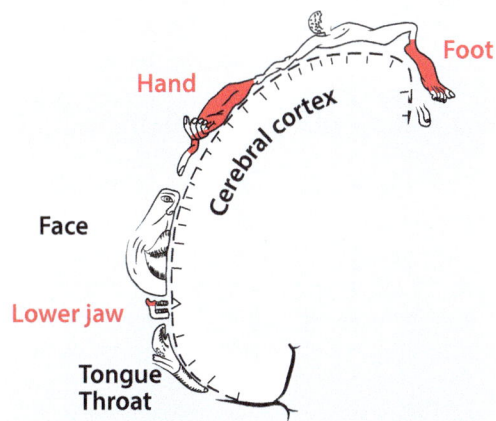

Representation of the different areas of the body in the cerebral cortex. Large areas are particularly well represented, i.e. they receive a particularly large number of pain nerve fibers from the periphery. The larger an area is represented in the brain, the denser the supply of pain nerve fibers in the corresponding area. The areas that are particularly affected by rheumatoid arthritis are marked in red here.

◘ **Fig. 5.2** Representation of the various body areas in the cerebral cortex changes in function. However, pain can also be triggered in the spinal cord itself or in the brain with appropriate stimulation of the centers.

In the chronic course, the sensitization mentioned above leads to a change in the character of the pain and to a fixation, whereby the initial triggering stimulus can lose more and more importance. It can happen that a previously painful foot, but amputated for some time, still causes pain, although this should no longer be the case after the foot has been removed. This is also called phantom pain. This is because the pathways for the amputated foot in the spinal cord and brain are still present, and the previous pain has become permanently imprinted there; sensitization has occurred in the spinal cord and brain. The affected individuals cannot get rid of the pain, even though the foot has long since been severed.

If this sensitization is favorable in acute pain, it is very problematic in chronic pain. If a rose thorn penetrates the skin and causes acute pain, sensitization is useful to provide relief and wound care. In the context of chronic pain, however, sensitization is a problem because it unnecessarily amplifies and maintains pain. Once again, it becomes clear that principles of acute pain have been preserved in the course of evolutionary history. Unfortunately, the same principles are also applied in chronic pain, even though it is not useful there.

5.6 Electric Shock, Pain, and Energy Expenditure

To estimate the relationship between pain on the one hand and increased energy expenditure on the other, one must use suitable methods of inducing pain in human studies that are ethically justifiable. Consider the famous experiments by Stanley Milgram, who conducted a horrifying psychological experiment at Yale University in 1961 (see Infobox "Explanation") to test the willingness to obey by applying pain stimuli from one test person to another. Therefore, pain experiments require a very special examination by the responsible ethics committees.

The Milgram Experiment

A test person, who acted as a teacher, gave a student electric shocks when a task was not performed correctly. However, the student was an actor, and when he received feigned electric shocks, he screamed loudly. Over the course of the experiment, the test person (teacher) increased the current strength at the request of an experimenter due to an accumulation of errors, causing the student to scream louder. In this way, the test persons (the teachers) administered very high electric shocks to their actor "students" because they did not want to resist the instructions of the experimenter and showed exaggerated obedience.

The experiment was so significant at the time because it was seen that even seemingly harmless test persons were ready for drastic actions at any time.

In a study in Nanjing, China, in 2013, the experimenters gave a group of freshly operated patients a painkiller for 3 days and then from day 3 either a placebo or a painkiller. They then examined the increase in pain and energy expenditure in the two groups in the days after the operation. As one would expect, they observed increased pain perception from day 3 to the end of the experiment on day 7 in the placebo-treated patients. They also determined the increased energy expenditure per day. The placebo-treated group needed on average 940 kJ (225 kcal) more energy per day than the group with painkillers. The groups were very homogeneously selected, so the increased energy expenditure was almost certainly due to the increased pain. Other studies roughly confirm the increased energy expenditure with postoperative pain.

In another experiment at the University of Aarhus in Denmark in 2009, electric shocks were applied to the abdominal skin near the navel. The test person set the level of pain themselves and applied the electric shock themselves. However, the pain was supposed to be severe. On a subjective scale from 0 [low] to 10 [high], the value 8 was to be reached. Anyone who could not reach it did not have to participate. In this experiment, the same test persons were subjected to three different scenarios:
- 1) with electric shocks,
- 2) with electric shocks and anaesthetization of the abdominal skin, and
- 3) without electric shocks and without anaesthetization of the abdominal skin.

When comparing the different scenarios, it was found that the people with the electric shocks without anaesthetization consumed about 69% more energy than the same people in the context of the other scenarios. Extrapolated to the day, they consumed 12,409 kJ (2964 kcal), while only about 7787 kJ (1860 kcal) were consumed under the two control situations. Furthermore, the researchers found that in the group with electric shocks and without anaesthetization, the blood levels of the stress hormones increased significantly.

This controlled experiment clearly shows that pain is associated with a significant increase in energy expenditure. In addition, the stress hormones cortisol, noradrenaline, and adrenaline are released, and a situation is created that strongly inhibits the effect of the storage hormone insulin. The inhibition of insulin action was clearly demonstrated by the authors. In this way, energy-rich substrates such as glucose are released from the stores or newly produced in the liver. All findings of this Danish working group show that the high energy expenditure is caused by immediate metabolic changes. These changes clearly show that above all, more glucose is made available as an energy-rich substrate. This is a typical immediate reaction of the stress axes.

Similar studies have not been conducted in patients with chronic pain because they are not ethically justifiable. However, based on the above findings, it can be assumed that chronic pain can also be associated with a significantly increased energy expenditure, especially when the pain is not well controlled or not treated at all.

5.7 Heat, Cold and Energy Expenditure

When we look at ◘ Fig. 5.1, we recognize that heat and cold stimuli are also transmitted via these nerve fibers. Heat situations such as during a sauna visit are known to significantly increase energy expenditure. A Finnish study showed that a sauna situation with 80°C dry heat for one hour a day and over 7 days increased the basal metabolic rate by 25–33%. At the same time, there was an increase in heart rate, which can be seen as a sign of the activation of the known stress axes (sympathetic nervous system).

Nevertheless, the sauna can be healthy if it is used in moderation and if the person does not have any cardiovascular problems, high blood pressure or arteriosclerosis. The sauna can lead to better monitoring of the body by the immune system, because the activation of the stress axes contributes to an increase in the migration of immune cells in the vascular system and in the rest of the body. Especially in winter, this increased "surveillance measure" can provide additional protection against infectious agents.

Heat and cold increase energy expenditure when the so-called thermoneutral range is left. The thermoneutral range is between 25 and 30 degrees Celsius for unclothed individuals. In this range, we need the least energy for "heating" and for "cooling". Below 25 degrees we need more energy for "heating" and above 30 degrees for "cooling" (sweating, ion pumps). Our nerve fibers recognize this range with finely tuned temperature sensors at the nerve endings described above and cause the energy expenditure, either for heating or cooling.

In a nutshell

- The sensation of pain was not abolished in our evolutionary history, but was retained to learn avoidance strategies and to quickly bring about appropriate help actions.
- Mechanical, thermal and chemical triggers of pain are distinguished.
- The chemical triggers that activate the pain receptor include
  - Acid,
  - Bacterial components,
  - Danger signals from immune cells,
  - Cytokines,
  - Pepper extract,
  - Body's own substances of the type of pepper extract,
  - Hormones and
  - Nerve messengers like noradrenaline.
- The recognition of the inflammatory state or the lack of oxygen in the tissue is ensured by pain nerve fibers.
- The face, the tongue, throat, hands and feet are most densely supplied with pain nerve fibers. There, an inflammatory situation can be recognized particularly well ("sixth sense").
- Pain causes significantly increased energy expenditure. In a Danish study, energy expenditure increased by 69%; from 10,000 kJ (2388 kcal) to 16,900 kJ (4036 kcal).
- Heat and cold increase energy expenditure when the thermoneutral range of 25–30 degrees Celsius is left. Heat and cold are also measured via the nerve fibers.

References

Basbaum AI, Bautista DM, Scherrer G, Julius D (2009) Cellular and molecular mechanisms of pain. Cell 139:267–841

Bluthe RM, Walter V, Parnet P, Laye S, Lestage J, Verrier D, Poole S, Stenning BE, Kelley KW, Dantzer R (1994) Lipopolysaccharide induces sickness behaviour in rats by a vagal mediated mechanism. C R Acad Sci III 317:499–503

Dhaka A, Uzzell V, Dubin AE, Mathur J, Petrus M, Bandell M, Patapoutian A (2009) TRPV1 is activated by both acidic and basic pH. J Neurosci 29:153–158

Hensellek S, Brell P, Schaible HG, Brauer R, Segond von Banchet G (2007) The cytokine TNFalpha increases the proportion of DRG neurones expressing the TRPV1 receptor via the TNFR1 receptor and ERK activation. Mol Cell Neurosci 36:381–391

Holland-Fischer P, Greisen J, Grofte T, Jensen TS, Hansen PO, Vilstrup H (2009) Increased energy expenditure and glucose oxidation during acute nontraumatic skin pain in humans. Eur J Anaesthesiol 26:311–317

Leppaluoto J, Tuominen M, Vaananen A, Karpakka J, Vuori J (1986) Some cardiovascular and metabolic effects of repeated sauna bathing. Acta Physiol Scand 128:77–781

Schaible HG, Ebersberger A, von Banchet GS (2002) Mechanisms of pain in arthritis. Ann NY Acad Sci 966:343–354

Schaible HG, von Banchet GS, Boettger MK, Brauer R, Gajda M, Richter F, Hensellek S, Brenn D, Natura G (2010) The role of proinflammatory cytokines in the generation and maintenance of joint pain. Ann N Y Acad Sci 60–69

Watkins LR, Goehler LE, Relton JK, Tartaglia N, Silbert L, Martin D, Maier SF (1995) Blockade of interleukin-1 induced hyperthermia by subdiaphragmatic vagotomy: evidence for vagal mediation of immune-brain communication. Neurosci Lett 183:27–31

Xu Z, Li Y, Wang J, Li J (2013) Effect of postoperative analgesia on energy metabolism and role of cyclooxygenase-2 inhibitors for postoperative pain management after abdominal surgery in adults. Clin J Pain 29:570–576

Psychological Stress and Energy

Contents

6.1   What is Stress? – 84

6.2   Acute Stress—Sport as a Model – 84

6.3   Chronic Stress is Unhealthy – 85

6.4   Chronic Stress at Work – 86

6.5   Stressful Double Hits – 87

6.6   Psychological Stress Causes Increased Energy Expenditure – 87

6.7   Dementia and Heart Disease Increase Energy Expenditure – 88

References – 89

6.1 What is Stress?

When experts are asked what exactly stress is, they almost uniformly respond that they themselves are not really clear about it. In experiments, there are many different bodily reactions to psychological stress, and no one knows exactly what the most important and thus the most representative response is. But when the scientific community is not clear about the representative answer, everyone uses their favorite tool. One uses psychological instruments such as questionnaires, another physical responses such as sweat secretion or heart rate, another investigator uses symptoms such as insomnia, gastrointestinal problems, headaches, others use blood values such as interleukin-6, etc.

Furthermore, people react very differently to stress, as the recognition of stressful situations, the processing of stress in the brain, the assessment of stress and the handling of or response to stress can vary greatly. This also depends heavily on the experimental circumstance, as stress can be triggered in many different ways.

A popular method of acutely inducing stress in humans is an unprepared speech in front of an "important" examination committee, where the performance can allegedly decide on professional development. The test is called *Trier Social Stress Test* (TSST), because it was invented at the University of Trier, Germany. This test is used worldwide today.

Stress can also be triggered by lack of space, for example under solitary confinement conditions or in a stationary elevator. Here, psychologists have not yet been able to agree on a uniform procedure for investigating stress, resulting in very different responses.

An integrated concept regarding psychological stress suggests that stress represents a constellation of events, where initially a stimulus must exist (stressor), which triggers a response in the brain (stress recognition) and a fight-or-flight reaction in the body (stress response). This interpretation seems to strongly refer to an acute event, and chronic stress with various triggers is probably not fully represented in this way. Similar to inflammation and pain, a distinction is made between acute and chronic events.

6.2 Acute Stress—Sport as a Model

Acute stress is less harmful and even useful, while chronic stress can cause illness. Our ancestors were confronted with acute stress in our evolutionary history, and so it can be understood that many mechanisms in the context of acute stress were preserved (positively selected) during evolution. Acute stress prepares us for difficult situations. In the case of acute stress, there is a short-term activation of the stress axes, and this is recognized by the increase in stress hormones such as cortisol, adrenaline and noradrenaline. Acute stress is also often associated with a stimulation of the immune system, which was referred to in ▶ Chap. 3 as "mutual immediate assistance (of the brain for the immune system)". Interleukin-6 is a typical signal that then tends to increase slightly (see ◘ Fig. 4.2). In the case of stress, various types of immune cells are primarily released into the blood circulation. Acute stress can therefore be defined via the hormones of the stress axis or the accompanying co-reaction of the immune system.

Physical exercise is often used as a model to simulate acute stress. Here, the fight-and-flight reaction is simulated, although the acute mental tension is missing in moderate sports. It has been proven many times that regular moderate exercise reduces the risk of cancer, slows the progression of cancer diseases and reduces the overall mortality from various ailments such as cardiovascular diseases. It has also been shown that moderate physical activity prevents infectious diseases, even if life was otherwise described as quite stressful.

6.3 Chronic Stress is Unhealthy

The situation is quite different with chronic stress. Here, the brain's stress response becomes fatigued because chronic stress represents a constant strain. Secondly, the response of the stress axes is weaker, which must be understood as fatigue of the stress axes, the adrenal gland, and the sympathetic nervous system. Thirdly, we recognize that the immune system is inhibited by chronic stress. The suppression of the immune system must be understood as a typical reaction of the selfish brain towards the immune system. Furthermore, many unfavorable behaviors such as smoking, poor nutrition, or lack of exercise occur. This behavior must be seen as a faulty reward response of the permanently exhausted brain.

Intense and prolonged sport was used as a model for chronic stress. With intense and long physical activity or sport under extreme conditions, there is a chronic strain. Here, the individual becomes susceptible to infectious diseases, but paradoxically also to cardiovascular diseases such as arteriosclerosis and heart attack. In an article from March 27, 2009, DIE WELT reported about a marathon runner who had died, probably due to a lingering herpes infection and who started training too soon. Therefore, sports are prohibited in case of fever and cough.

Another form of chronic stress was addressed in ▶ Chap. 4 "Inflammation and Energy". It is about the chronic stress in the family care of a dementia patient, for example in Alzheimer's disease, or in the care of disabled people. This form of stress was referred to as *Caregiver-Stress*. This is truly a very difficult situation, as often years of self-sacrificing work is done, which is associated with a higher risk for various diseases. It has been proven that family caregivers have a higher risk of depression, cardiovascular diseases, and arteriosclerosis and show increased inflammatory activity (see ◘ Fig. 4.2).

But the dementia patient himself also suffers from his situation. The increasing development of dementia with restrictions of perception or a disabling physical illness is perceived as chronic stress by the affected patient. If dementia leads to a loss of the usual control over daily life, for example due to loss of temporal and spatial orientation, this can mean significant chronic stress with increased physical activity and sleep disorders. This overwhelming situation is then perceived as stressful by the affected person himself and the family caregivers. Since this situation often lasts for years, it is chronic continuous stress for the affected person and the caregivers.

Events in childhood such as neglect, sexual abuse, acts of violence, impoverish-ment, disputes and divorce of parents, death of a parent, serious illness of a parent, mental illness in parents and similar serious, long-term influences also represent a chronic continuous strain. These childhood adverse experiences are perceived as chronic stress and means changes in reprogramming the stress axes. Later sequelae such as depression, other psychiatric diseases, and chronic inflammatory diseases show the long-term influence, which could be demonstrated in many studies (see a newer book of the author of 2023 mentioned in the Reference List). This was par-ticularly found in the childhood form of chronic arthritis.

Physical and psychological traumas such as war experiences, weather-related disasters, rape, death of a close person and similar events in adulthood are per-ceived as chronic stress. A so-called post-traumatic stress syndrome can develop as a result. Chronic traumas also include suffering such as cancer, heart attack, heart failure, or autoimmune diseases.

According to Charles Cooley—an American sociologist (1864–1929)—people are social beings. Loneliness is therefore particularly perceived as very stressful, es-pecially by the elderly. The connection between loneliness and subsequent problems such as depression, sleep disorders, heart attack, stroke, accumulation of infections and increased inflammation situation is known; often this leads to increased mor-tality. Loneliness is chronic stress for many people.

6.4 Chronic Stress at Work

Finally, let's point out the chronic stress at work. Who hasn't experienced this by himself/herself? Many complications at work are perceived as stressful, where it is actually about the personally perceived level of stress.

The most serious problem, however, is the imbalance between performance on the one hand and reward on the other. Some people often take on very high obliga-tions without being properly rewarded for it. It is called *"organizational injustice"* or *"effort-reward imbalance"* . This imbalance between performance and reward forms a serious chronic stress signal, leading to depression, heart attacks, high blood pres-sure, obesity, stroke, and other subsequent diseases.

Sometimes it is absurd how employers exploit the willingness of employees to perform without getting a picture of the development of subsequent problems of this chronic stress. This often happens when these superiors have gone through sim-ilar careers and have not gained insight into stress-related problems in themselves or others. Our work culture is gradually improving, occupational physicians in large companies are increasingly paying attention, but the process is particularly slow in this country – Germany – with its high work ethic. This is regrettable because the follow-up costs, especially of depressive and other mental illnesses, are enormous and these problems are steadily on the rise..

At some point, the general public will spend more money on the subsequent problems than the general public previously took in the form of taxes, contribu-tions, etc. from the successful work of those affected. At the latest then and better now, we must start to consistently ensure a healthy working climate. This must be an active and deliberate political process.

6.5 Stressful Double Hits

There are certainly many more aspects of chronic stress exposure that have not been listed here. So this collection makes no claim to completeness. However, one thing should be mentioned, and that is additive and synergistic effects. When chronic stressors come together, effects on health can intensify in the sense of an addition or beyond as a synergism (◘ Table 6.1).

We can call this coming together of two factors "double hit". It has been clearly demonstrated that the combination of depressive mood and an additional inflammatory disease significantly exacerbates the problem. This can go so far that a manifest depression develops where previously only possible depressive symptoms or chronic stress exposure could have been spoken of. This coming together of several stressful elements is repeatedly discussed in this book as a "double hit".

6.6 Psychological Stress Causes Increased Energy Expenditure

Let's return to the main topic of the book and ask ourselves whether acute or chronic stress leads to higher energy expenditure. The answer is obvious. Both acute and chronic stress situations increase energy expenditure. The connection is particularly clear for acute stressful life events, as they involve a fight-or-flight response, which always goes hand in hand with high energy expenditure. We discussed that sport can be used as a model for acute stress, and it is quite obvious that this means more energy expenditure.

But even in acute psychological stress tests like the *Trier Social Stress Test*, there is a significant increase in energy expenditure. In this particular case of psychological stress, a Lübeck working group led by Achim Peters observed an overcompensation of voluntary energy intake after the test in the form of tasty snacks. Overcompensation means that too many energy-rich substrates were consumed in relation to the test-induced energy expenditure. The 10-minute test led to a stress-related increase in intake of 26% of the total daily energy required by the brain, which was about 571 kJ (137 kcal) after the test. This would be as if the brain had been active for more than 6 hours instead of 10 minutes. If this is always the case, we need to protect ourselves from stress-related events because of the risk of weight gain.

In fact, about 40% of people gain weight under stress, 40% lose weight, and 20% remain the same (the golden mean). We will discuss weight changes in more detail

◘ **Table 6.1** What is addition and what is synergism?

Addition	Synergism
You have two factors A and B, which can exert the two effects designated **Effect (A)** and **Effect (B)** on a biological system.	You have two factors A and B, which can exert the two effects designated **Effect (A)** and **Effect (B)** on a biological system.
In an **additive effect**, the total effect is equal to the sum of the individual effects: Total effect = Effect (A) + Effect (B)	In a **synergistic effect**, the total effect is greater than the sum of the individual effects: Total effect > Effect (A) + Effect (B)

in Part III of the book. There, it will be explained why some people gain weight under stress and others lose weight.

Let's consider chronic stress, for example, as long-term intense sport. Of course, this form of physical activity leads to higher energy expenditure over long periods of time. But also family *Caregivers* have higher energy expenditure, as could be demonstrated in family members caring for children. It was found that *Caregivers* with a high heart rate and high oxygen consumption as a measure of energy expenditure found this work particularly stressful.

It was also shown in these individuals that the heart rate is well linked to the increased energy expenditure. This finding points to the importance of the sympathetic nervous system as an energy provider during stress. Furthermore, the mere increase in physical work for *Caregivers* is a significant factor for increased energy expenditure. In a Japanese study, the energy expenditure during the usual working time was about 7482 kJ (1787 kcal) in 8 hours. Add the energy expenditure of a minimal work performance for the remaining 16 hours and you end up with about 12,482 kJ (2981 kcal). This is the energy expenditure for moderate to heavy work.

Even in children with a family tragedy or chronic abuse, there is an increased energy expenditure with simultaneously lower energy intake, which can best be observed in growth disorders. If a child falls below the 70% mark of the expected body weight or the predicted body size, hospital admission should be considered and the psychosocial environment should be checked in any case. Interestingly, these children sleep less, which can explain part of the increased energy expenditure.

People with post-traumatic stress disorder, have a similar sleep deficit. This inevitably leads to higher energy expenditure.

6.7 Dementia and Heart Disease Increase Energy Expenditure

Patients with Parkinson's disease and dementia can have increased energy expenditure, especially when the disease is long-lasting, of higher severity, and there is higher muscular activity. These Parkinson's patients often also lose weight, which represents a negative prognostic signal. Weight loss is also common in Alzheimer's patients, even though enough energy is consumed. This is particularly true for physically highly active Alzheimer's patients. This also suggests a higher energy expenditure in this chronic stress of dementia. In mice with Alzheimer's disease, an increased energy expenditure of about 24% per day was observed.

In another disease associated with dementia, Huntington's disease, weight loss and increased energy expenditure are also a known phenomenon. Here, an 11–20% increased energy expenditure was measured, and mice with this disease also show increased energy consumption. Patients with Huntington's disease exhibit increased voluntary, but also involuntary physical activity.

We can summarize that dementia—a chronic stressful disease—is associated with increased energy expenditure and often with weight loss, when there is higher physical activity and sleep problems.

But also patients with a chronic physical disease, who do not have a strong inflammation, can show an increased energy expenditure. Thus, in a large study on patients with heart failure, a higher energy expenditure than in normal persons was measured. The basal metabolic rate in these patients was 7319 kJ (1748 kcal) per day and in normal persons 6611 kJ (1579 kcal) per day. It was noted in ▪ Table 1.1in ▶ Chap. 1 that this energy expenditure at absolute rest is about 7500 kJ (1791 kcal) per day. The values given here are somewhat smaller, so one must assume people with a lighter body structure.

Patients with severe heart failure and muscle loss showed no increased energy expenditure because they protect their energy stores. Also, children with a congenital heart defect show a 35% increased energy expenditure per day compared to healthy children. This imbalance can then lead to growth disorders.

In a Nutshell

- One distinguishes between acute and chronic stress. Acute stress can be healthy and is best represented by short-term, moderate physical activity.
- Acute stress is associated with a mild activation of the immune system (a higher immune surveillance). We called this the "mutual immediate assistance of the brain for the immune system and vice versa."
- Chronic stress is disease-causing. Intense and long-lasting sport can be used as a model.
- Other conditions and diseases are also experienced as chronically stressful:
  - caregiving for family members (*Caregiver stress*),
  - dementing diseases like Parkinson's,
  - childhood adverse experiences (example: severe illness and death of a parent),
  - severe stressful life events in adulthood (example: war experiences),
  - chronic disease like heart failure,
  - loneliness, especially in old age,
  - workplace stress
  - and many others.
- When chronic stressors come together, effects on health can add up or even mutually reinforce each other in the sense of a synergy (▪ Table 6.1).
- Acute and chronic stress increase daily energy expenditures.
- Energy expenditures increase by about 10–35% above the normal level in chronic stress; so from 10,000 kJ (2388 kcal) per day to 11,000 kJ–13,500 kJ (2627–3224 kcal) per day.

References

Dhabhar FS (2014) Effects of stress on immune function: the good, the bad, and the beautiful. Immunol Res 58:193–210

Eijsvogels TM, Fernandez AB, Thompson PD (2016) Are There Deleterious Cardiac Effects of Acute and Chronic Endurance Exercise? Physiol Rev 96:99–125

Gaba AM, Zhang K, Marder K, Moskowitz CB, Werner P, Boozer CN (2005) Energy balance in early-stage Huntington disease. Am J Clin Nutr 81:1335–1341

Gavrieli A, Farr OM, Davis CR, Crowell JA, Mantzoros CS (2015) Early life adversity and/or posttraumatic stress disorder severity are associated with poor diet quality, including consumption of trans fatty acids, and fewer hours of resting or sleeping in a US middle-aged population: A cross-sectional and prospective study. Metabolism 64:1597–1610

Hawkley LC, Cacioppo JT (2010) Loneliness matters: a theoretical and empirical review of consequences and mechanisms. Ann Behav Med 40:218–227

Hitze B, Hubold C, van DR, Schlichting K, Lehnert H, Entringer S, Peters A (2010) How the selfish brain organizes its supply and demand. Front Neuroenergetics 2:7–17

Kiecolt-Glaser JK, Derry HM, Fagundes CP (2015) Inflammation: depression fans the flames and feasts on the heat. Am J Psychiatry 172:1075–1091

Straub RH (2023). Early Trauma as the Origin of Chronic Inflammation: A Psychoneuroimmunological Perspective. Springer Nature, Berlin.

6

Other Energy-Consuming Situations

Contents

7.1   Sleep Problems—Sleep Apnea – 92

7.2   Chronic Smoldering Infections – 92

7.3   Fear and Anxiety – 94

7.4   6 Cigarettes per Day – 95

References – 96

7.1 **Sleep Problems—Sleep Apnea**

In our younger years, a person can sleep without interruptions for up to 12 hours, which can significantly change over the course of life. During sleep, we require about 25–30% less energy, so a person with a total daily expenditure of 10,000 kJ (2388 kcal) needs approximately 2373 kJ (567 kcal) during the 8 hours of sleep and about 7627 kJ (1821 kcal) during the remaining 16 hours of wakefulness. Thus, we clearly recognize that sleep conserves energy expenditure because the muscles are relaxed and the brain operates at a slightly lower level. Sleep disorders, which are associated with increased wakefulness, lead to increases in energy expenditure.

It has been shown that people with chronic insomnia have an increased energy expenditure of 10–15% compared to healthy normal individuals and consequently suffer from daytime fatigue. Furthermore, these patients showed a higher body temperature and an increased heart rate as signs of increased activity of the sympathetic nervous system. This was substantiated by elevated blood levels of noradrenaline. Remember that noradrenaline and adrenaline are the neurotransmitters of the sympathetic nervous system. Furthermore, higher blood levels of the other stress hormone cortisol from the adrenal cortex were detected.

All these points suggest an increased activity of the stress axes. They are responsible for energy provision.

In addition, chronic insomnia also leads to increased appetite, which can be explained by the increased need for energy. However, if overcompensation were to occur, as we have already described in the psychological stress test, the energy intake could be significantly higher than the energy expenditure caused by lack of sleep. The consequence would be unwanted weight gain.

Since sleep disorders actually lead to an increase in diabetes and obesity, there is much to suggest overcompensation and other disturbances of the energy balance. A recent study showed that energy intake exceeds the increased energy expenditure. This increased energy intake then particularly occurs later in the evening after dinner. This evening overcompensation has now been confirmed by other authors.

In patients with sleep apnea syndrome, who experience nocturnal breathing pauses and pronounced daytime fatigue, the overall energy expenditure is increased. It was found that energy expenditures can increase by 30%. This would mean an increase from 10,000 kJ (2388 kcal) to 13,000 kJ (3104 kcal) per day for a patient with a sedentary life style. In individuals who respond well to therapeutic nocturnal positive airway pressure ventilation, the energy expenditure can be reduced to the normal value. In children, this additional energy expenditure seems to be less significant.

So it is exactly as one would expect with reduced sleep: there is a higher energy expenditure in sleep disorders. However, this increased energy expenditure is more than compensated for by a high energy intake, so that over time the body weight can steadily increase.

7.2 **Chronic Smoldering Infections**

Even though we no longer suffer from the chronic infectious diseases of earlier times such as tuberculosis or leprosy in today's highly developed countries, there are still chronic infections that can affect the life of one or another person. This is particularly the case when people get older and the immune system changes. This is a typical phenomenon in stressful life events—just think of cold sores, which are often reactivated under stress (when skiing with strong sunlight). But it is also the case with all serious diseases such as AIDS or various forms of cancer, where the immune system is affected.

There are chronic infections with cytomegalovirus in humans. Initially, the cytomegalovirus causes minor disease symptoms, fever, swollen lymph nodes, and mild liver involvement. Later, the presence of the cytomegalovirus is hardly noticed anymore. But since it belongs to the herpes viruses, it can, like the herpes viruses, stay in our body for a long time. It can then reappear under unfavorable conditions, like cold sores. The presence of the cytomegalovirus has been linked to heart attack, especially when there is a higher inflammation situation at the same time. Cold sores in susceptible people carrying the virus have also been linked to chronic inflammatory problems.

The well-known Epstein-Barr virus causes the acute disease of so-called infectious mononucleosis with severe lymph node and spleen swelling, fever, throat inflammation, and liver involvement. It is a very infectious disease that usually heals quickly and without complications. However, the Epstein-Barr virus remains in the body for life in 98% of people. Under unfavorable conditions, it can become active again and cause inflammation problems. The presence of the Epstein-Barr virus has been linked to various diseases such as autoimmune diseases but also to chronic fatigue syndrome.

We also know of protracted infections with chlamydia, bacteria that affect the upper respiratory tract and can cause bronchitis and pneumonia. These bacteria are usually well controlled and can only become active under certain circumstances and cause the known problems in the bronchi and lungs.

In the stomach, the chronic presence of Helicobacter pylori, a spiral-shaped bacterium, is known. This bacterium can cause a chronic infection of the stomach in some people. It has been linked to the development of stomach ulcers, duodenal ulcers, but also stomach cancer. These complications illustrate the long-term activity of these bacteria, although those affected often notice little of this chronic smoldering infection.

There are also various hepatitis viruses that can cause chronic liver inflammation. Sometimes these hepatitis viruses are in the body for a long time without causing major problems. The affected individuals are called "chronic virus carriers".

The list of infections mentioned here is certainly not complete, but it illustrates the problem of chronic smoldering infection. Chronic infections are associated with a higher inflammation situation and, thus, also with a slightly increased energy expenditure after activation.

Since the probability of suffering from the various infectious diseases mentioned increases with age, these problems are likely to become greater with increasing age. Over the course of life, one accumulates various pathogens, some of which one can no longer get rid of. The usual antibiotics do not help with the viruses, and even after successful antibiotic treatment, there is a risk of relapse with the bacteria, as described for Helicobacter. Since the infectious agents interact with the immune system, a chronic, mild inflammation can take place largely unnoticed.

Even though individuals with such chronic infections have rarely been studied in terms of energy expenditure, the example of Hepatitis C—a chronic liver inflammation caused by the Hepatitis C virus—may be an example of the problem. In these patients, it was shown that the chronic virus carrier with good liver function, without liver cirrhosis and without obvious disease symptoms, had an increased energy expenditure per day at absolute rest of 6409 kJ (1530 kcal) compared to the healthy control group of the same size (165 cm) and with similar body weight (68 kg) with 5842 kJ (1395 kcal). Thus, the chronic smoldering infection leads to an additional energy expenditure of about 10%. For a person with a sedentary life style and an energy expenditure of 10,000 kJ (2388 kcal), that would be about 1000 kJ (239 kcal) more per day.

It has already been shown above that the simultaneous occurrence of several cytokines, as described in the Swiss experiment with the bacterial components, leads to an additive or even synergistic increase in energy expenditure. This is likely to be the case with two or even three different chronic smoldering infections, although this has never been investigated. This situation could also be called a "double hit".

7.3 Fear and Anxiety

Fears cause a stressful feeling, which is why they could have been mentioned under psychological stress (e.g., exam stress and exam anxiety). Fears are even positive when they are short-lived and represent adequate responses to typical stimuli. Fears protect the affected person from dangerous situations. Fears have not been abolished in the course of evolution, but have been conserved (positively selected) in order to better cope with dangers. However, the fear should not become too great, as it otherwise makes action impossible.

One distinguishes a situation-dependent fear (*"state anxiety"*) from the relatively stable character trait of anxiety (*"trait anxiety"*). If one has an exaggerated fear, then one also speaks of an anxiety disorder, which may require therapy. On a scale from 0 to 100, situation-dependent fear and also character-dependent anxiety can occur in very different degrees. Both forms of fear can be quantitatively recorded with questionnaires.

Typical responses to fear are activation of the sympathetic nervous system and the cortisol stress axis, dilation of the pupils (sympathetic activation), increased blood pressure and heart rate (sympathetic activation), faster and shallower breathing, sweating (sympathetic activation), trembling, inhibition of the gastrointestinal tract (sympathetic activation), sometimes nausea and others. From these symptoms, we quickly recognize that many reactions are controlled by the stress axis of the sympathetic nervous system. If the sympathetic nervous system plays such an important role, it would not be surprising if situation-dependent fear or anxiety were associated with a higher energy expenditure.

A research team studied college students at a university in the northwest of the USA. All had to fill out a questionnaire on fear/anxiety. Then they compared those students without fear/anxiety with those individuals with high fear/anxiety in terms of basal metabolic rate (lying in bed at rest, awake, fasting). It turned out that the students in the high-anxiety group spent about 703 kJ (168 kcal) more per day than the students in the low-anxiety group. Now, 703 kJ (168 kcal) is not little, considering that the resting immune system requires about 1600 kJ (382 kcal) per day. Thus, increased fear/anxiety alone takes up almost half of the daily consumption of the quiescent immune system. What will this be like in patients with a psychiatrically diagnosed anxiety disorder?

Furthermore, it could be shown that individuals with high anxiety have a lower physical activity, so it can be assumed that the higher basal energy expenditure is compensated by a lower energy expenditure with less physical activity.

7.4 6 Cigarettes per Day

Do you know the smoker who used to smoke quite a lot, and after quitting cigarettes, gained a significant amount of weight? As reported by the Federal Centre for Health Education, according to a study by the German Cancer Research Centre, four out of five smokers gain 4–5 kg within the first two years after quitting. At least five mechanisms are held responsible for this:

- 1) Metabolism slows down after quitting (lower energy expenditure).
- 2) The feeling of hunger/appetite increases.
- 3) Sweets and snacks are consumed more frequently as a substitute.
- 4) The gut flora undergoes a change in composition after quitting smoking (new microbes extract more energy from food).
- 5) Bowel emptying slows down.

Regarding point 4, scientists have shown that a change in gut bacteria is responsible for the increased energy intake after quitting. After quitting smoking, different strains of bacteria in the gut come more and more to the fore, and these then contribute to a better absorption of energy components from food.

At this point, we also recognize an influence of evolutionary processes, as the coexistence of "host" and bacteria underwent a long common evolutionary history. Thus, in the non-smoking host under conditions of lower food availability, those types of bacteria that caused improved digestion and a higher provision of energy-rich components were particularly promoted.

Furthermore, a detailed study of 236 participants examined to what extent smoking increases total energy expenditure. Indeed, smoking more than 6 cigarettes per day increases energy expenditure in men by 1250 kJ (298 kcal) and in women by 678 kJ (162 kcal). Higher amounts of cigarettes were not tested, but it is conceivable that this can be increased even further. The higher energy expenditure in a smoker is associated with increased heart rate and increased blood pressure as signs of stimulation of the sympathetic nervous system (stress axis). This gives smokers the kick (adrenaline junkies), which, in addition to the taste experience, also positively stimulates the brain and body. It is therefore not surprising that for centuries after the introduction of tobacco in Europe, it was assumed that smoking was healthy and invigorating. Only the large population-based studies from the USA in the 1950s made the various subsequent problems of smoking clear, especially lung cancer.

In a nutshell

— Good sleep conserves energy reserves, and sleep problems lead to increased energy expenditure.
— Sleep problems increase energy intake in response to the increased energy expenditure caused by lack of sleep, and too much energy is consumed (overcompensation is discussed in ▶ Chap. 14 in relation to weight gain).
— In sleep apnea syndrome, energy expenditures can increase by 30%.
— Over the course of life, we accumulate chronic smoldering infections. Using the example of chronic liver inflammation caused by the Hepatitis C virus, we clearly see significantly increased energy expenditure in the order of 1000 kJ (239 kcal) per day.
— Situation-dependent anxiety and character-based anxiety increase the basal metabolic rate per day by about 10%, or 703 kJ (168 kcal).
— Smoking leads to increased energy expenditure. There is a dose-effect relationship that could be described as: the more cigarettes, the more energy expenditure.
— Smoking also leads to a change in gut flora compared to non-smokers, which induces worse digestion and also inferior provision of energy-rich components from the food.

References

Astrup A, Toubro S, Cannon S, Hein P, Breum L, Madsen J (1990) Caffeine: a double-blind, placebo-controlled study of its thermogenic, metabolic, and cardiovascular effects in healthy volunteers. Am J Clin Nutr 51:759–767

Black AE, Coward WA, Cole TJ, Prentice AM (1996) Human energy expenditure in affluent societies: an analysis of 574 doubly-labelled water measurements. Eur J Clin Nutr 50:72–92

Blaxter K (1989) Energy metabolism in animals and man. Cambridge University Press, Cambridge New York New Rochelle Melbourne Sydney

Bonnet MH, Arand DL (1995) 24-Hour metabolic rate in insomniacs and matched normal sleepers. Sleep 18:581–588

Fekete K, Boutou AK, Pitsiou G, Chavouzis N, Pataka A, Athanasiou I, Ilonidis G, Kontakiotis T, Argyropoulou P, Kioumis I (2016) Resting energy expenditure in OSAS: the impact of a single CPAP application. Sleep Breath 20:121–128

Gonseth S, Dugas L, Viswanathan B, Forrester T, Lambert V, Plange-Rhule J, Durazo-Arvizu R, Luke A, Schoeller DA, Bovet P (2014) Association between smoking and total energy expenditure in a multi-country study. Nutr Metab (London) 11:48–11

Judice PB, Matias CN, Santos DA, Magalhaes JP, Hamilton MT, Sardinha LB, Silva AM (2013) Caffeine intake, short bouts of physical activity, and energy expenditure: a double-blind randomized crossover trial. PLoS One 8:e68936

Markwald RR, Melanson EL, Smith MR, Higgins J, Perreault L, Eckel RH, Wright KP, Jr (2013) Impact of insufficient sleep on total daily energy expenditure, food intake, and weight gain. Proc Natl Acad Sci USA 110:5695–5700

Muhlestein JB, Horne BD, Carlquist JF, Madsen TE, Bair TL, Pearson RR, Anderson JL (2000) Cytomegalovirus seropositivity and C-reactive protein have independent and combined predictive value for mortality in patients with angiographically demonstrated coronary artery disease. Circulation 102:1917–1923

Patterson RE, Emond JA, Natarajan L, Wesseling-Perry K, Kolonel LN, Jardack P, Ancoli-Israel S, Arab L (2014) Short sleep duration is associated with higher energy intake and expenditure among African-American and non-Hispanic white adults. J Nutr 144:461–466

Piche T, Schneider SM, Tran A, Benzaken S, Rampal P, Hebuterne X (2000) Resting energy expenditure in chronic hepatitis C. J Hepatol 33:623–627

Rolfe DF, Brown GC (1997) Cellular energy utilization and molecular origin of standard metabolic rate in mammals. Physiol Rev 77:731–758

Schmidt WD, O'Connor PJ, Cochrane JB, Cantwell M (1996) Resting metabolic rate is influenced by anxiety in college men. J Appl Physiol (1985) 80:638–642

Van Cauter E, Spiegel K, Tasali E, Leproult R (2008) Metabolic consequences of sleep and sleep loss. Sleep Med 9 Suppl 1:S23–S28

What Does Increased Energy Expenditure Mean for the Body?

Contents

8.1   Energy Expenditure in Aging – 101

8.2   Energy Expenditure is Hereditary – 103

8.3   Energy Situation During Aging with Additional Energy Expenditures – 104

References – 107

Let's take a closer look at the energy expenditure of a healthy young person again. In a resting body position in bed, the energy expenditure is minimal. It is also called the basal metabolic rate (BMR in ◘ Fig. 8.1).

When we consume food, we expend a small amount of energy after eating, which is due to the digestive processes. It is also called the food-induced energy expenditure ("Food" in ◘ Fig. 8.1). However, much less energy is expended than we take in through eating and drinking (only about 10% of it).

Then there is the portion of energy expenditure due to physical activity, which we call activity-related energy expenditure (AEE in ◘ Fig. 8.1). The brain

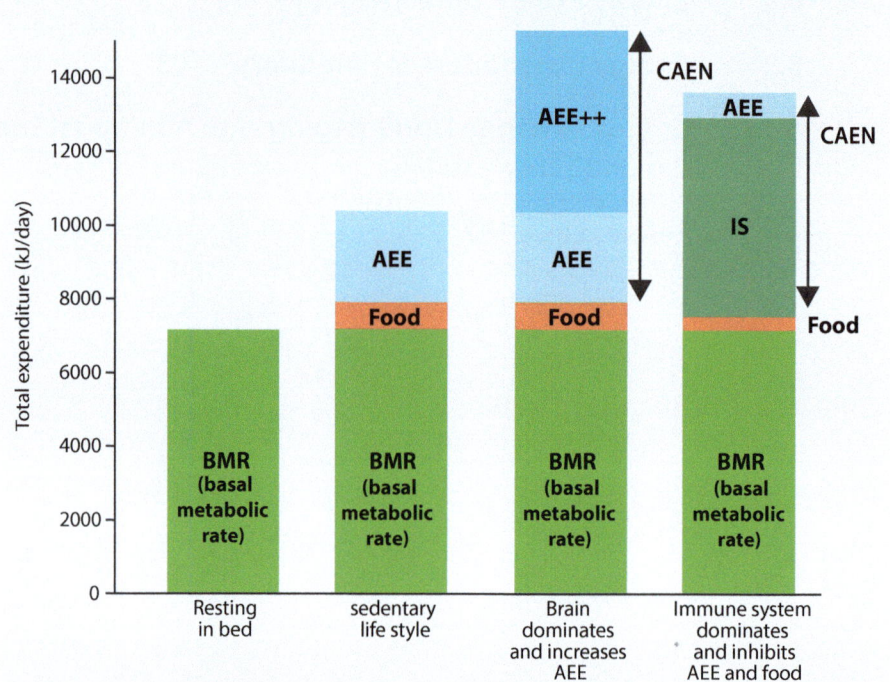

Energy expenditure under different conditions.
- Energy expenditure at rest without food (1st column from the left, corresponds to the basal metabolic rate, BMR
- with seated posture and eating (2nd column from left),
- with an increase in activity by the selfish brain (3rd column from the left)
- when the selfish immune system is activated (4th column from the left).

It can be seen that when the activity of the selfish immune system increases, both "eating" and activity-related energy expenditure (AEE) are significantly reduced.

Abbreviations:

AEE = activity-related energy expenditure

AEE++ = activity-related additional expenditure over and above a normal activity-related energy expenditure

CAEN = "controllable amount of energy", the negotiable energy expenditure over and above the basal metabolic rate (negotiating partners are the brain and immune system, chap. 3)

BMR=basal metabolic rate

IS = additional energy expenditure by an activated immune system above the normal level

◘ **Fig. 8.1**   Energy expenditure under various conditions

dominates this activity-related energy expenditure, as physical activity and muscle work are initiated by the brain. The brain can increase this expenditure at any time under certain circumstances (AEE++ in ◘ Fig. 8.1). However, due to the selfish behavior of the immune system, the energy expenditure of the immune system can also be greatly increased (IS in ◘ Fig. 8.1). Under the conditions of increased expenditure by the selfish immune system, the energy expenditure through physical activity (AEE) is restricted. The same is true when the energy expenditures are increased by other factors mentioned in ▶ Chaps. 5–7. This primarily comes at the expense of voluntary physical activity.

When several energy-consuming factors come together, effects on health can be additive or even synergistic. These would then also be "double hits" or even "multiple hits". For example, it has been shown that the combination of depressive mood and additional inflammatory disease significantly exacerbates the problems. This combination of several stressful energy expenditures either restricts voluntary physical and mental activity or the immune system.

It is indeed a struggle for resources, which can be bitterly fought among selfish participants.

8.1 Energy Expenditure in Aging

To better understand the situation in aging, we need to consider the energy situation during the healthy aging process. Excellent studies have been conducted by various working groups, providing us with a very good picture of the healthy aging human (◘ Fig. 8.2).

During healthy aging, the basal metabolic rate, the energy expenditure caused by physical activity, and the energy expenditure caused by food intake continuously decrease from the age of 50. As we age, the proportion of time spent with low-intensity physical activity increases. At the same time, the fat-free mass (muscles, bones, internal organs, etc.) steadily decreases (green line in ◘ Fig. 8.2). In parallel, the fat mass in relation to body weight steadily increases (red line in ◘ Fig. 8.2).

When fat-free mass decreases and fat mass increases, a mismatch between muscle and fat tissue occurs. This results in less physical activity and better storage of energy components. This is a spontaneously increasing problem that can also become a vicious cycle, ending in high fat mass. This is not exactly what one dreams of.

Many important works on this topic come from Klaas Westerterp from Maastricht in the Netherlands. For example, his group observed that in people under 50, total physical activity and thus energy expenditure increase with training, as the young person under 50 maintains the same level of activity for the rest of the day despite extra training. In people over 50, total physical activity and energy expenditure do not increase with extra training, as more time is spent at rest outside of training. The usual level of activity is reduced.

It is also important to know that the young person under 50 compensates for the extra energy expenditure with extra food during training. The same does not apply to people over 50. Strangely, people over 50 consume the same amount of energy

8

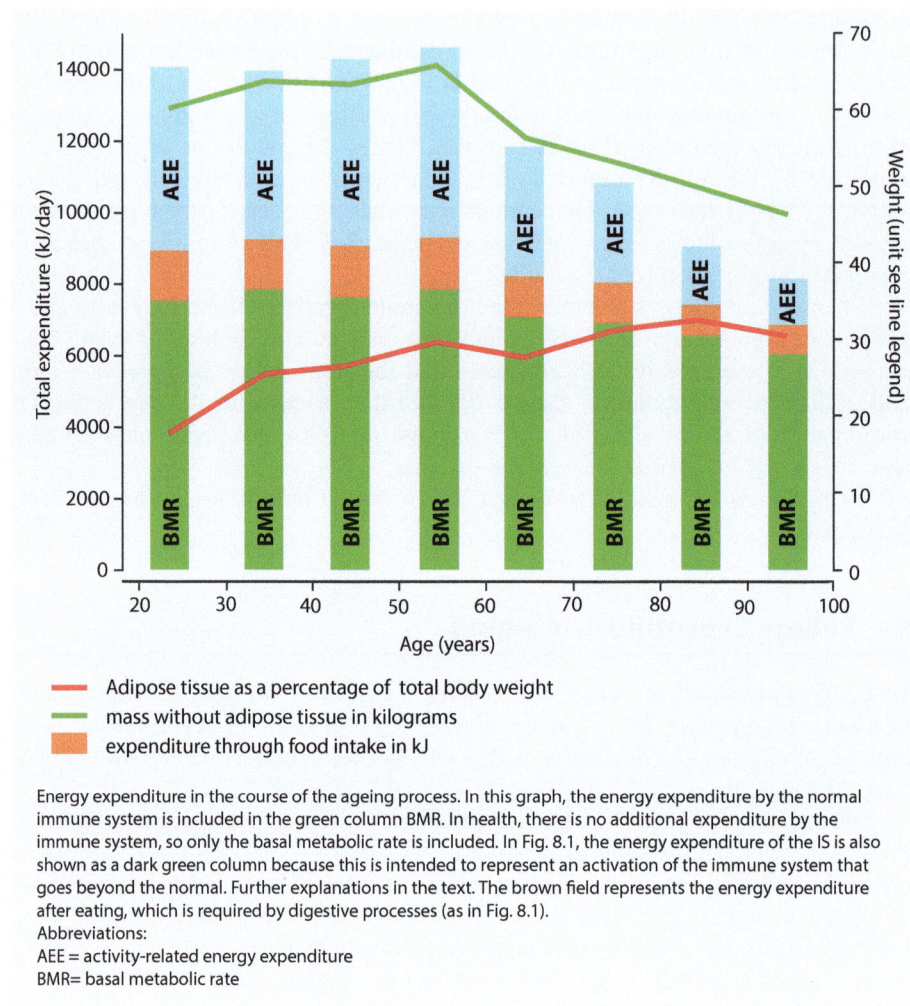

Energy expenditure in the course of the ageing process. In this graph, the energy expenditure by the normal immune system is included in the green column BMR. In health, there is no additional expenditure by the immune system, so only the basal metabolic rate is included. In Fig. 8.1, the energy expenditure of the IS is also shown as a dark green column because this is intended to represent an activation of the immune system that goes beyond the normal. Further explanations in the text. The brown field represents the energy expenditure after eating, which is required by digestive processes (as in Fig. 8.1).
Abbreviations:
AEE = activity-related energy expenditure
BMR= basal metabolic rate

Fig. 8.2   Energy expenditure during the aging process. (Data from Speakman and Westerterp 2010)

with or without training. Probably, with shrinking internal organs, one cannot eat as much over 50 (this will be explained in the next two paragraphs).

In a very fascinating experiment by Westerterp's working group, young and older people with an average age of 24 and 56 years respectively had to intensively mountain climb in the high mountains for 10 days. The average daily distance was 21 km, and the average height to climb was 1160 m per day, so it can be assumed that both groups were quite well trained. The total daily energy expenditure was 21,500 kJ (5135 kcal), close to the absorption limit in the intestine (■ Table 1.1 in ▶ Chap. 1). With these high energy expenditures, it was observed that the young people could almost compensate for the energy expenditure with a large food intake of 19,200 kJ (4586 kcal). The group of older participants, who had the same energy expenditures, on average only consumed 15,200 kJ (3583 kcal) through food. This discrepancy led to significant weight loss in the older, but not in the young mountaineers.

In ▪ Fig. 8.2, it was shown that in old age the fat-free mass decreases. This primarily includes muscles, bones, and internal organs. It is impressive that especially the internal organs such as the liver and gastrointestinal tract become smaller. This also explains why the older participants in the mountain tour consumed less food. On average, the older participants' food intake per day was 4000 kJ (955 kcal) lower than that of the young mountaineers. The consequence of very high energy expenditure in old age is weight loss.

It should be added that these experiments with mountaineers represent an extreme form of energy consumption, as we usually consume and expend significantly less energy.

8.2 Energy Expenditure is Hereditary

It is also interesting that the propensity for physical activity is hereditary. Thus, there are people who are born athletes and spend their entire lives with a very high level of physical activity. On the other hand, there are people who always show a low level of physical activity and prefer sedentary jobs.

In a study with identical twins with an average age of 25 years, physical activity was examined more closely. The twins lived in different places. It was thus shown that the identical twins exhibited a very similar level of physical activity. If one identical twin was highly active, so was the other. The percentage of hereditary influence on physical activity was about 75%. This is an extremely high percentage in inheritance studies.

And then there is a particularly interesting phenomenon in the course of the healthy aging process. People who show a high level of physical activity in their younger years gain more fat weight during aging than those who show a sedentary, less active lifestyle in their younger years. Physically active people are used to consuming larger amounts of food compared to less active people. Of course, they also need a higher energy intake with an active lifestyle. Perhaps they also have a larger liver and a larger gastrointestinal tract that allows this intake. So if the young active people can take in more food, they would have to adjust their food intake with decreasing physical activity in old age, and that's exactly what they don't do. The excess food intake then leads to larger fat deposits, because what is taken in excess is stored. In the end, sedentary, less active people may be better off because they are used to taking in little food.

At this point, we must once again turn to evolutionary medicine. Isn't it interesting that the aging process, with regard to these energy issues, begins precisely from the age of 50 (see ▪ Fig. 8.2)? The 50th year of life is very critical for both women and men because the activity of many sex hormones decreases significantly (menopause in women and andropause in men). Since reproduction also significantly decreases or stops at the same time, it can be assumed that hardly any genes and dependent mechanisms for a happy and healthy aging were positively selected in the course of evolutionary history after the age of 50.

If someone is very physically and mentally active in old age, it must be assumed that the necessary genes and mechanisms were conserved for youth and the first adult years—for reproduction and fight-or-flight reaction etc.— in the ancestors of this person over generations. It may well be that we possess some favorable mechanisms in old age, but they were not specifically selected for this aging process. On the other hand, it may also be that we inherited very positive genes from our ancestors for youth and the first adult years over hundreds of generations, which can be unfavorable in old age. This insight comes from evolutionary biologist George Christopher Williams from Charlotte, North Carolina, who recognized and described this connection as early as the 1950s. Williams was the co-founder of modern evolutionary medicine.

8.3 Energy Situation During Aging with Additional Energy Expenditures

Now there are constellations that do not go hand in hand with a chronic and severe inflammatory reaction, but consume a lot of energy. These factors were discussed in detail in ▶ Chaps. 4–7. These include chronic pain, chronic psychological stress, too much smoking, but also sleep problems, fear/anxiety, and chronic smoldering infections. This book certainly did not consider all points, and the reader may add his personal example of increased energy expenditure here.

Finally, it also becomes clear that combinations of the mentioned points cause an additional problem ("double hit"), which must all lead to resource conflicts. Since many of the mentioned factors increase during the aging process, this energy conflict becomes visible in old age, even if there is no severe chronic inflammation as in chronic autoimmune diseases. Even a slightly increased inflammatory situation is enough to create a problem together with the other simultaneously occurring factors.

In the last three decades, increasing studies have been conducted on large populations that illuminated the relationship between a slight inflammatory situation on the one hand and complications on the other. In this inflammatory situation, one cannot speak of a chronic inflammatory disease, as typically much higher inflammation values are found there. The first studies on this were conducted with the erythrocyte sedimentation rate, then with the C-reactive protein, and finally also with interleukin-6. All mentioned parameters represent inflammation and are associated with increased energy expenditure. They did not increase very strongly in old age, as shown in ▪ Fig. 4.2.

Over time, a clear correlation has been found between these only slightly elevated inflammation factors, which were measured many years before the event, and an increased risk in old age for the following disease situations:

- Heart attack,
- Stroke,
- High blood pressure,
- Diabetes in old age,
- Blood clots,
- Bone loss (osteoporosis),
- Dementia,
- Depression,
- Macular degeneration and
- Colon cancer.

One can therefore assume that there is also a correlation between slightly elevated inflammation and increased mortality.

In this respect, it becomes apparent that a long-term mild inflammation, which is associated with increased energy expenditure, is also associated with an increased risk of disease. This is particularly true when additional unwanted factors such as chronic pain, chronic psychological stress, excessive smoking, but also sleep problems, anxiety/fear, and chronic smoldering infections are also present ("double hit").

But what happens under the conditions of additional unwanted energy expenditure during aging? For this, we need to take a closer look at ◘ Fig. 8.3 below. There, a fictitious energy expenditure was introduced in dark green color and labeled IS+. IS stands for immune system, and the plus sign refers to the other unwanted factors leading to additional expenditures such as chronic pain, chronic psychological

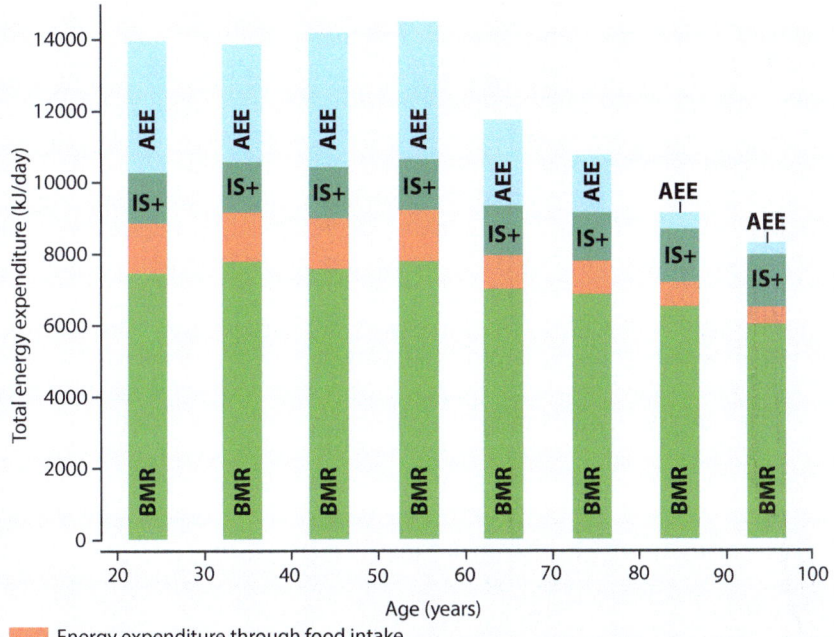

■ Energy expenditure through food intake

Energy expenditure in the course of the ageing process with simultaneous additional unwanted energy expenditure. Additional unwanted energy expenditure comes from an activated immune system (IS) and others such as chronic pain, chronic psychological stress, excessive smoking, sleep problems, fear/anxiety and chronic smoldering infections. It is evident that these additional unwanted energy expenditures have the greatest impact on physical activity (AEE decreases visibly). Due to the age-related decline in AEE, the problem becomes particularly pronounced from around the age of 50. As in Fig. 8.1, the additional energy expenditure is also shown as a dark green column (called IS+).
Abbreviations:
AEE = activity-related energy expenditure
BMR = basal metabolic rate
IS+ = IS = additional energy expenditure by an activated immune system above the normal level

◘ **Fig. 8.3**   Energy expenditure during the aging process with simultaneous additional unwanted energy expenditure

stress, excessive smoking, sleep problems, anxiety/fearfulness, and chronic smoldering infections in the sense of a "double hit" or "multiple hit."

With the introduction of the additional unwanted energy consumption IS+, the expenditure for voluntary physical activity (AEE) decreases at the same time. Now it was already very noticeable in ◘ Fig. 8.2 that especially the fat-free mass (muscles, bones, internal organs, etc.) decreases during aging, but the fat mass relatively increases. Under a constellation with increased energy expenditure due to the above-mentioned unwanted factors from ► Chaps. 4–7 (chronic pain, chronic psychological stress, excessive smoking, sleep problems, anxiety/fear, and chronic smoldering infections) and simultaneous restriction of physical activity, this process is significantly promoted. The reduction of physical activity while maintaining the youthful food intake inevitably leads to too high energy intake. Physical inactivity plays a causal role in the development of overweight and obesity and the associated secondary diseases.

If we now look at the results in ◘ Fig. 8.3 (age 80–90 years), this is comparable to the situation of a chronic inflammatory disease in younger years. In severe inflammation, the selfish attitude of the immune system leads to the constellation shown in ◘ Fig. 8.1 (4th column from the left). After all, in chronic inflammatory disease, there is a decrease in voluntary physical activity even in young years. This decrease in physical activity is then even more pronounced in older people with a chronic inflammatory disease.

If physical activity is restricted in a chronic inflammatory disease, this results in a higher risk of cardiovascular diseases, as recently shown in a large Canadian study of over 12,000 normal individuals and over 1000 patients with rheumatoid arthritis.

It can be summarized that the situation in older people with various unwanted factors leading to high energy expenditure (► Chaps. 4–7) is similar to the situation in chronic inflammatory diseases. However, in the case of chronic inflammatory disease, the selfishness of the immune system comes much more to the fore, which is why the problems become visible already in youth or middle adulthood.

With all these considerations, it also becomes understandable that the subsequent problems, which are dealt with in the third part of the book, are comparable in chronic inflammatory disease and during aging.

In a nutshell

- Energy expenditure arises from the body's basal metabolic rate, a small energy consumption caused by food intake, and energy expenditure caused by physical activity.
- The energy consumption caused by food intake corresponds to about 10% of the energy taken in through food.
- When multiple energy-consuming processes come together, problems can intensify additively or synergistically. Example: Symptoms of a mental upset during a simultaneous infectious disease can lead to depression.
- In healthy aging, the basal metabolic rate and the energy expenditure caused by physical activity (AEE) continuously decrease only from the age of 50.
- Furthermore, the fat mass relative to body weight steadily increases, and the fat-free mass (e.g., muscles, internal organs, bones, and others) steadily decreases.

- Genes and dependent mechanisms were not positively selected for a long-lasting aging process associated with well-being in evolutionary history (after reproductive time, from the age of 50).
- If additional unwanted energy-consuming factors are added during aging, the energy expenditure through voluntary physical activity decreases. This particularly affects people from the age of 50. Even normal people move less from the age of 50, but still eat like in their younger years (therefore they get fatter).
- The situation during aging with additional unwanted energy-consuming factors can then correspond to the situation of a chronic inflammatory disease. The key point is the lack of voluntary physical and mental activity.

References

Black AE, Coward WA, Cole TJ, Prentice AM (1996) Human energy expenditure in affluent societies: an analysis of 574 doubly-labelled water measurements. Eur J Clin Nutr 50:72–92

Elia M, Ritz P, Stubbs RJ (2000) Total energy expenditure in the elderly. Eur J Clin Nutr 54 Suppl 3:S92–103

Manini TM (2010) Energy expenditure and aging. Ageing Res Rev 9:1–11

Munsterman T, Takken T, Wittink H (2012) Are persons with rheumatoid arthritis deconditioned? A review of physical activity and aerobic capacity. BMC Musculoskelet Disord 13:202–213

Ramsey JJ, Harper ME, Weindruch R (2000) Restriction of energy intake, energy expenditure, and aging. Free Radic Biol Med 29:946–968

Schieir O, Hogg-Johnson S, Glazier RH, Badley EM (2016) Sex Variations in the Effects of Arthritis and Activity Limitation on First Heart Disease Event Occurrence in the Canadian General Population: Results From the Longitudinal National Population Health Survey. Arthritis Care Res (Hoboken) 68:811–888

Speakman JR, Westerterp KR (2010) Associations between energy demands, physical activity, and body composition in adult humans between 18 and 96 y of age. Am J Clin Nutr 92:826–834

From Energy and Evolution to Symptom

Before the sequelae of misguided energy expenditure and lack of voluntary physical activity are discussed in detail in this part of the book, the sequelae or symptoms will now be listed here. The list does not claim to be complete, and the readers may expand it themselves. It only contains the most severe signs of disease and symptoms that physicians and patients observe in chronic inflammatory diseases, but also during aging. The numbering is based on the chapter numbers.

- 9 – Daytime Fatigue and Depression
- 10 – Sleep Disorders and Circadian Symptoms
- 11 – Loss of Appetite, Malnutrition and Undernutrition
- 12 – Muscle Loss
- 13 – Bone Loss
- 14 – Weight Changes (increase and decrease)
- 15 – Insulin Resistance and Hyperinsulinemia
- 16 – Decreasing Libido, Lower Fertility
- 17 – High activity of the sympathetic nervous system and high blood pressure; in contrast: low activity of the parasympathetic nervous system
- 18 – Increased Blood Clotting
- 19 – Stress Worsens Inflammation, and Inflammation Alters Stress Tolerance

In the following chapters, these signs of disease and symptoms will now be dealt with individually, with a focus on the chronic inflammatory disease and parallel consideration of aging.

Daytime Fatigue and Depression

Contents

9.1   Sickness Behavior in Chronic Inflammatory
       Disease – 112

9.2   Daytime Fatigue and Depression in Old Age – 114

       References – 115

9.1 Sickness Behavior in Chronic Inflammatory Disease

Over the past three decades, the relationship between inflammation in the periphery (e.g., during infection) and in the brain and the so-called *"Sickness behavior"* (we have already become acquainted with it) has been investigated. The pioneering work was done by the research group led by Robert Dantzer from Bordeaux. *Sickness behavior* is understood as the sum of various symptoms such as

- Discomfort,
- Daytime fatigue, exhaustion,
- Lack of drive,
- Increased feeling of cold,
- Muscle pain, joint pain,
- Loss of appetite,
- Anxiety,
- Depressive feelings,
- Withdrawal into familiar safe areas and
- "Lack of energy."

The last symptom in particular strongly indicates the connection with the actual energy supply in the physical sense of this book.

An extreme situation of *Sickness behavior* can be constant sleep. During sleep, large amounts of energy can be saved, as shown in ◘ Fig. 9.1.

The lower part of ◘ Fig. 9.1 shows the brain's glucose consumption, which is much lower during sleep (◘ Fig. 9.1b). It should be added that the energy saved by the resting state of the muscles is much greater than the saving by the sleeping brain. Energy expenditure during sleep is about 25–30% lower than when awake. We have learned that during infections, the energy conflict of the immune system with that of the brain and muscles becomes important (► Chap. 3, "Brain and Immune System—Two Competing Realms").

Sickness behavior has been preserved (positively selected) during evolution, and it serves to save energy by reducing physical and mental activity. If it is a short episode during an infectious disease, the advantage of this *Sickness behavior* quickly becomes clear. Each of us has experienced a similar situation when we were bedridden with the flu. The saved energy is used for the active immune system. However, if the situation persists for some reason, this *Sickness behavior* can easily become a permanent state.

Robert Dantzer from Bordeaux even suggests that in susceptible individuals, major depression can develop from *Sickness behavior*. Because in principle, the *Sickness behavior* described above only differs from depression in terms of chronicity. In certain forms of depression, other brain-specific factors probably need to be added independently of inflammation.

However, scientists from Atlanta led by Andy Miller were able to show that even the continuous administration of a cytokine in the therapy of a viral hepatitis can trigger depression. This suggests that some forms of depression probably arise largely on the basis of a smoldering inflammatory situation, if this situation persists long enough. In that observation from Atlanta, an antidepressant could reduce the problems, which speaks for the "authenticity" of the depression.

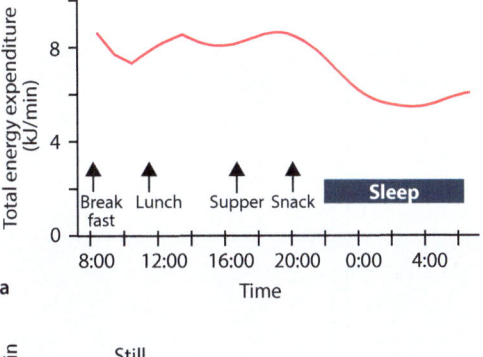

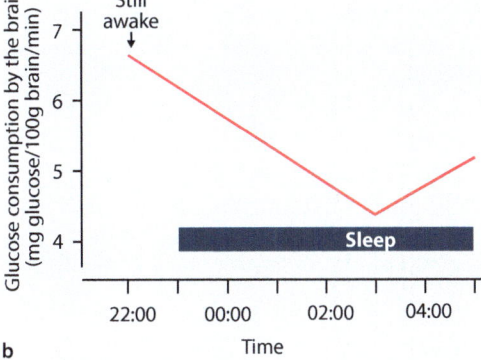

Saving energy through sleep.
a Here, the total energy expenditure in kJ/min is plotted over the course of the day in healthy people. During the phase of wakefulness - especially after meals - energy expenditure is relatively constant at around 8 kJ/min. With the onset of sleep, the output is reduced to around 4.2 kJ/min. It is almost halved compared to the waking state.
b The consumption of glucose by the brain is plotted against the time. The brain consumes about 6.5 mg of glucose per 100 g of brain tissue per minute when awake. This value decreases significantly after falling asleep and reaches its minimum at around 3 am.

■ **Fig. 9.1** a, b Energy saving through sleep. **a** Total energy expenditure, **b** Glucose consumption by the brain. (Data from Ravussin et al. 1986; Boyle et al. 1994)

In chronic inflammatory diseases, it has been clearly established in the last three decades that many patients suffer from chronic daytime fatigue. However, if you check more closely, many people not only have daytime fatigue, but they also suffer from many of the symptoms of the above-mentioned *Sickness behavior*. This is explained using the example of the chronic inflammatory disease rheumatoid arthritis. Interestingly, in this disease, the inflammation activity measured in the blood does not correlate well with daytime fatigue (e.g., using the following inflammation factors: erythrocyte sedimentation rate, C-reactive protein, or interleukin-6). Daytime fatigue is much more strongly associated with the presence of chronic pain. Individuals with a high number of painful joints suffer more from daytime fatigue.

Pain can significantly contribute to increased energy expenditure alongside inflammation. Indeed, the aforementioned Danish study involving the electrical stimulation of the abdominal skin showed that daily energy expenditure can increase by 69% from 10,000 kJ (2388 kcal) to 16,900 kJ (4036 kcal) due to pain (▶ Chap. 5 "Pain and Energy"). For daytime fatigue, in the chronic inflammatory disease of rheumatoid arthritis, pain signals are more important than the inflammation measurable in the blood. However, since the pain in this chronic inflammatory disease is triggered by local inflammatory processes, it is difficult to distinguish between energy expenditure due to an activated immune system—i.e., inflammation—and energy expenditure due to pain.

Regardless, the energy conflict, as depicted in ◘ Fig. 8.1, becomes apparent when the immune system is activated in the context of chronic inflammatory diseases. The consequence of the energy conflict is daytime fatigue and, in some individuals, depression and other symptoms of *Sickness behavior*. This daytime fatigue ultimately leads to reduced physical activity with all the ensuing problems.

But what does the situation look like during aging?

9.2 Daytime Fatigue and Depression in Old Age

We have learned that the normal aging process is accompanied by a slightly increased inflammatory constellation. However, the inflammation is of minor extent compared to the chronic inflammatory disease of rheumatoid arthritis (◘ Fig. 4.2). In Part II "Energy Expenditure in the Spotlight" (▶ Chaps. 4–7) of the book, the various situations with unwanted energy expenditure that increasingly occur with age were presented. These include chronic pain, chronic psychological stress, excessive smoking, sleep problems, anxiety/fear, and chronic smoldering infections. The problems can also add up or work synergistically ("double hit"), so that significant amounts of energy are not available for the selfish brain and thus for healthy physical/mental activity, nor for a selfish immune system and thus for adequate infection defense.

Often, one or more triggers are at the beginning of the chain of effects. Infections, injuries, stroke, short-term high stress load, onset of a chronic disease, cell death in the brain in Alzheimer's disease, or others can start the process, disrupt the regulation, and lead to an energy shortage.

This energy shortage can then express itself in old age very similarly to a chronic inflammatory disease as daytime fatigue, especially as sleep problems often exist. If the unwanted energy expenditure caused by the various age-related problems mentioned is significant, the development of *Sickness behavior* up to depression is a possible scenario. It has been proven that the frequency of depression increases with age. Associated with this problem are psychological stress for the affected person and for the family environment, increased costs in the healthcare system, further diseases, and increased mortality due to suicide. In addition, this constellation is associated with further sleep problems, so that a vicious circle can arise here, which then has to be broken with external help.

One thing is certain: The increased unwanted energy expenditure during aging is associated with reduced voluntary physical and mental activity. This constellation was depicted in ▣ Fig. 8.3. Reduced physical and mental activity is then a significant risk factor for further complications.

References

Boyle PJ, Scott JC, Krentz AJ, Nagy RJ, Comstock E, Hoffman C (1994) Diminished brain glucose metabolism is a significant determinant for falling rates of systemic glucose utilization during sleep in normal humans. J Clin Invest 93:529–535

Buysse DJ (2004) Insomnia, depression and aging. Assessing sleep and mood interactions in older adults. Geriatrics 59:47–51

Dantzer R, O'Connor JC, Freund GG, Johnson RW, Kelley KW (2008) From inflammation to sickness and depression: when the immune system subjugates the brain. Nat Rev Neurosci 9:46–56

Musselman DL, Lawson DH, Gumnick JF, Manatunga AK, Penna S, Goodkin RS, Greiner K, Nemeroff CB, Miller AH (2001) Paroxetine for the prevention of depression induced by high-dose interferon alfa. N Engl J Med 344:961–966

Ravussin E, Lillioja S, Anderson TE, Christin L, Bogardus C (1986) Determinants of 24-hour energy expenditure in man. Methods and results using a respiratory chamber. J Clin Invest 78:1568–1578

Sleep Disorders and Circadian Symptoms

Contents

10.1   How can Sleep be Studied? – 118

10.2   Sleep and Circadian Rhythms in Chronic Inflammatory Diseases – 119

10.3   Circadian Rhythm of Inflammation – 120

10.4   Sleep Problems in Old Age – 123

References – 124

10.1 How can Sleep be Studied?

With the development of brainwave measurement via electrodes on the scalp, a new era of sleep research began in the 1920s (called electroencephalography). Different sleep phases were gradually defined based on the voltage fluctuations on the scalp. Many voltage fluctuations per second (up to 30× per second, or 30 Hertz) or very few voltage fluctuations of only 1 Hertz can be found. The fewer the number of fluctuations per second, the deeper one sleeps. The extreme is the zero line without voltage fluctuations, as occurs in brain death.

The first classification of the different sleep phases dates back to 1968, which was revised in 2007. Sleep is divided into several phases. Thus, we speak
- of light sleep phase (stage 1) shortly after falling asleep,
- of deeper stage-2 sleep with muscle relaxation and lower body temperature, and
- of deep sleep (stage 3, previously also stage 4).

Overall, one spends 50% of the time in stage-2 sleep with muscle relaxation and lower body temperature, both of which contribute to energy saving during sleep.
- These three consecutive sleep phases are interrupted by so-called REM sleep phases. REM stands for *"rapid eye movement"*. The REM sleep phase is also called dream sleep because people awakened during this phase report their dreams. It is astonishing that we do not physically move (can't move) during this REM sleep phase, but experience a lot, and only the eyes wander aimlessly back and forth. At the same time, blood pressure, breathing, and heart rate increase significantly. In the early phase of the night, the REM sleep phases are short at 5–10 minutes. After that, the duration of REM sleep increases steadily until morning.

According to this classification, sleep stages 1–3 are also referred to as Non-REM sleep, because the eyes do not move. Stages 1–3 followed by REM sleep are repeated several times per night (5–7×), with sleep depth decreasing and REM phases increasing. A sleep cycle consisting of Non-REM sleep (stage 1–3) and REM sleep lasts about 90 minutes.

If one wants to study sleep, there are several auxiliary variables that can be considered during sleep. For example, one measures the time from lying down to falling asleep, the total sleep time in minutes, the total sleep time in relation to the observation time (it is called sleep efficiency and is given in percent), the length of the individual sleep stages in minutes, the length of the total REM sleep phase in minutes, the number of sleep cycles per night, and the wake times after falling asleep until the end of the observation time. This list is not complete, but it gives a good indication of the known sleep variables.

After sleeping, one can then ask about the recovery effect of sleep, the severity of daytime sleepiness, physical activity, or general motivation, which is usually queried using so-called visual analogue scales from 1–10. For example, the number 1 can mean little daytime sleepiness and the number 10 can mean strongest daytime sleepiness. The numbers in between indicate intermediate degrees of daytime sleepiness. Some very sophisticated questionnaires have been developed that can query several points at the same time.

With this prior knowledge, one can now check whether the sleep physiology and the positive effects of sleep in patients with chronic inflammatory diseases present differently compared to normal individuals.

10.2 Sleep and Circadian Rhythms in Chronic Inflammatory Diseases

In a study on patients with rheumatoid arthritis, a Berlin working group at the Charité examined the above-mentioned parameters before and after intensive therapy. It was shown that sleep efficiency improved after therapy, the total sleep duration became longer, and the deeper stage-2 sleep was more pronounced. In parallel, perceived daytime fatigue decreased and activity improved. However, the patients were significantly below the values of healthy normal individuals, i.e., they had more sleep problems.

We have learned that patients with chronic inflammatory disease expend more energy for an active immune system, and it is rightly asked why they do not sleep better than healthy normal individuals. Shouldn't they be more tired? Since inflammation is often associated with inflammatory pain, and since inflammatory pain is very often a nocturnal to early morning problem, this can play an important role. ◘ Figure 10.1 shows the relationship between daytime on one side and joint stiffness, pain, and physical dysfunction on the other side.

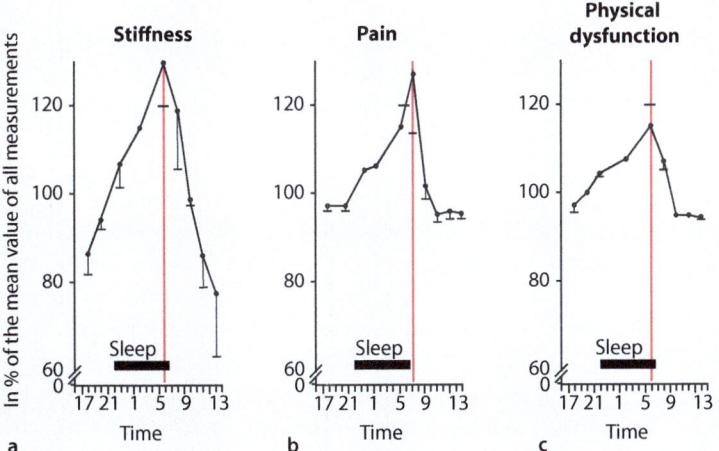

Circadian rhythm of joint stiffness, pain and physical dysfunction in rheumatoid arthritis. In the course of the day - also known as the circadian rhythm - problems increase, especially at night and in the morning hours. In all three examples, the problems start shortly after falling asleep. The maximum (red vertical line) is reached between 6 and 8 o'clock. This circadian symptomatology is characteristic of rheumatoid arthritis. Incidentally, physical weakness or dysfunction is measured by recording the time until a pellet is inserted into a tube. If a patient needs a lot of time for this seemingly simple task due to joint inflammation and stiffness, there is a clear physical dysfunction.

◘ **Fig. 10.1a–c** Circadian rhythm of joint stiffness, pain, and physical dysfunctions in rheumatoid arthritis. (Data from Straub and Cutolo 2007)

Patients with chronic inflammatory diseases often report nocturnal to early morning pain. It is characteristic of these diseases when an extraordinary pain is noticed at night, i.e., when one wakes up involuntarily due to pain. This necessarily disrupts sleep. Although one falls asleep again and again, the overall sleep takes on a different character by being broken up into pieces. It is then clear that the various sleep phases must change and the recovery effect is significantly reduced.

Sleep with a lower recovery effect leads to more pain, but also to higher inflammation. With lower pain thresholds, one suffers more from pain during the day, but especially at night. The nights can sometimes become long. This inevitably leads to higher energy expenditures due to the active immune system, the pain, and longer wakefulness.

10.3 Circadian Rhythm of Inflammation

Let's now look at the daily rhythm of our known inflammation factor Interleukin-6 in ◘ Fig. 10.2. This might give us a hint as to why the symptoms occur at night and in the early morning (as shown in ◘ Fig. 10.1). Inflammation can trigger and intensify pain.

Apparently, Interleukin-6 rises in the morning hours in patients with rheumatoid arthritis significantly higher than in normal individuals. Furthermore, other inflammation factors also increase in the morning hours (not shown in ◘ Fig. 10.2). If inflammation increases in the morning hours, then it is also understandable that pain increases in the morning hours and sleep is disturbed. One could now ask why the inflammation factor Interleukin-6 in ◘ Fig. 10.2 drops around 8 o'clock in normal individuals and around 10 o'clock in patients. What magical anti-inflammatory force is at work here?

To understand this, one must know that the stress axes, which we got to know in the first part of the book, also become active in the morning hours. These are the stress axis that produces cortisol from the adrenal cortex, and the sympathetic nervous system with noradrenaline (from sympathetic nerve fibers) and adrenaline (from the adrenal medulla). These three factors are the main players in the redistribution of energy, which is regulated by the brain (◘ Fig. 1.9 in ▶ Chap. 1).

In the morning hours, it is good if this energy redistribution takes place with these factors, because the brain and muscles need to be supplied with energy-rich substances. However, these are also the factors of the brain that suppress the immune system when the selfish brain claims the energy-rich substrates. In healthy individuals, the three factors have a parallel circadian rhythm (◘ Fig. 10.3).

The parallelism of the curves in ◘ Fig. 10.3 is astonishing and one immediately wonders if this has any significance. Indeed, it means mutual assistance! The hormones support each other in their effect in the sense of addition or beyond in the sense of synergism. This observation applies to the release of energy-rich substrates and to the inhibition of the immune system. If only one hormone is active, its effect is not as strong as when all three hormones cooperate.

Looking back at ◘ Figs. 10.1 and 10.2, it now also becomes clear that the inflammation in the morning hours is inhibited by the activity of the three hormones and thus the pain symptoms in the morning hours decrease again when the

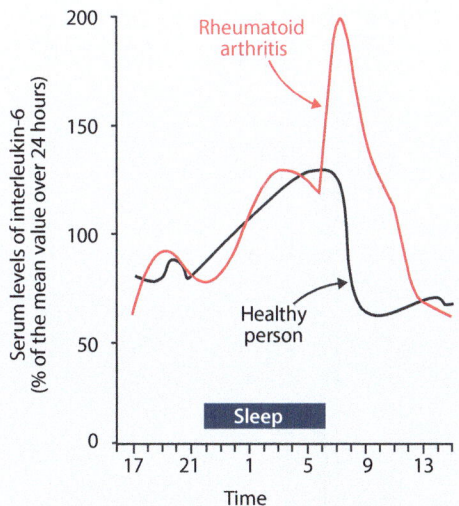

Circadian rhythm of interleukin-6 in patients with rheumatoid arthritis and healthy normal individuals. The red curve represents the data of the patients and the black curve the data of the normal persons. For better comparability, the values are given as a percentage of the daily mean value (100% value), around which they fluctuate. This circadian mean value is 2-4 pg interleukin-6 per milliliter of serum in normal persons, and it is around 20-40 pg/ml in patients with chronic inflammatory disease. You can see that the red curve rises higher than the black curve and that it falls 3 hours later in the morning.

■ **Fig. 10.2** Circadian rhythm of Interleukin-6 in patients with rheumatoid arthritis and healthy normal individuals. (Data from Straub and Cutolo 2007)

maximum has been exceeded. Conversely, it becomes clear that the minimum of the three hormones around 11 to 12 pm in ■ Fig. 10.3 must contribute to a nocturnal increase in the inflammation situation and the pain. The inflammation brake is missing.

In healthy individuals, the three factors from ■ Fig. 10.3 show parallel curves. In patients with chronic inflammatory diseases, the circadian curves of cortisol, adrenaline and noradrenaline are similar to those in healthy individuals, but the anti-inflammatory power of these hormones is not sufficient due to the strength of inflammation. The anti-inflammatory power of the hormones is also reduced by various degradation reactions in the immune cells.

As a result, the curves shown in ■ Fig. 10.2 for interleukin-6 look different. Inflammation dominates in chronic inflammatory diseases. This is particularly evident in the early phase without treatment. It can go so far that the parallel circadian rhythm of the three hormones from ■ Fig. 10.3 is abolished. In such a case, the anti-inflammatory cooperation of the three hormones is lost, which exacerbates

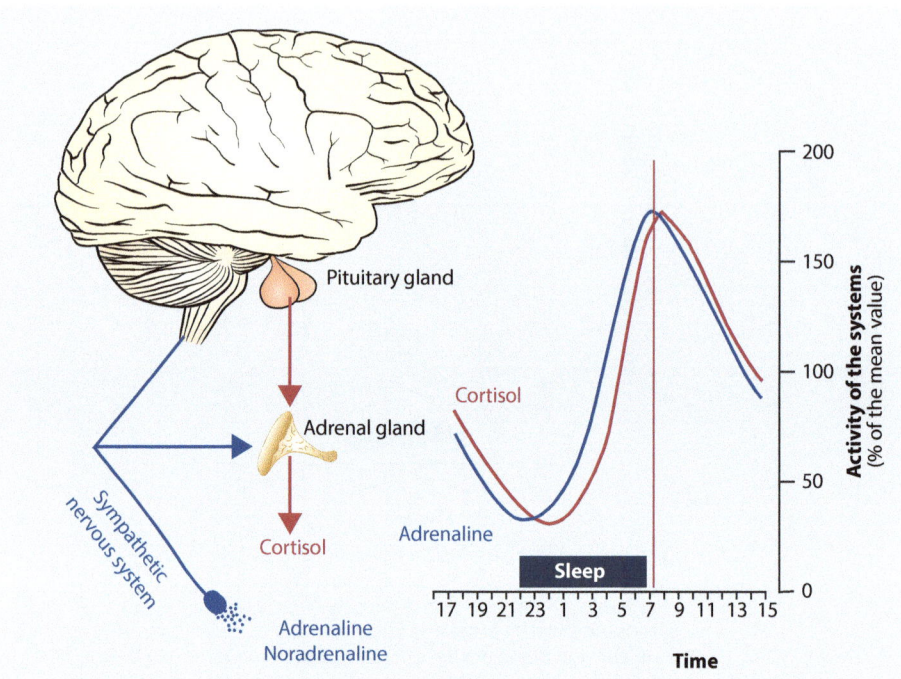

Circadian rhythm of cortisol and adrenaline/noradrenaline. Cortisol from the adrenal cortex, adrenaline from the adrenal medulla and noradrenaline from the sympathetic nerve fibers show a parallel rhythm with a maximum at around 7:15 a.m. and a minimum at 11 p.m. to midnight after falling asleep. These hormones release energy-rich substances, which can then be taken up by the brain. This includes glucose in particular. Furthermore, these hormones are also involved in inhibiting the activity of the immune system (Chapter 3 "Brain and immune system - two competing realms"). They are cooperative in terms of their functions, as they support each other.

■ **Fig. 10.3**   Circadian rhythm of cortisol and adrenaline/noradrenaline

the problem. As a result, the release of energy-rich substrates regulated by the brain is weaker, and the immune system now takes over the control of energy release through its own mechanisms, which were discussed in detail in ▶ Chap. 3 ("Brain and immune system—two competing realms").

Sleep disorders therefore occur due to nocturnal pain with increased inflammation. The disorder manifests itself in fragmented sleep, shorter sleep phases and less recovery effect. Since sleep disorders, inflammation and pain influence each other and all lead to increased energy expenditure, therapy in these patients must take into account all three elements (double and triple hit). Now one recognizes how complex the problem of higher unwanted energy expenditure is, and why the sole therapy of inflammation is not sufficient. The higher energy expenditures are responded to with daytime sleep and reduced physical and mental activity, thereby increasing the risks for cardiovascular diseases and metabolic diseases.

10.4 Sleep Problems in Old Age

During the aging process, sleep changes significantly. There is more insomnia (the majority complain about this) and more hypersomnia (too much sleep), as shown in 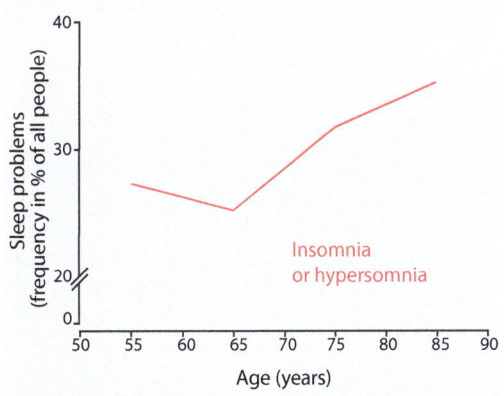 Fig. 10.4. Furthermore, a longer awake phase is observed from lying down to falling asleep, the total sleep time is reduced, and the sleep stages with deep sleep are shorter. Sleep in old age is increasingly fragmented by waking phases, which is then compensated by daytime sleep. The duration of the dreamy REM sleep phases decreases, the wakeability increases, and the perceived recovery effect is increasingly worse. If we now compare all this with the things in chronic inflammatory diseases, we recognize that the changes are very similar.

Where in chronic inflammatory diseases the immune system dominates and thus leads to increased energy expenditure and adjustment reactions, in old age the additional unwanted factors mentioned in Part II of the book "Energy Expenditure in the Spotlight" are relevant to cause very similar disturbances of energy expenditure and sleep. In normal aging, the nocturnal curve for inflammation using the example of interleukin-6 (■ Fig. 10.2) and the nocturnal curve for pain (■ Fig. 10.1) look very similar to those in chronic inflammatory diseases.

The typical problems that even a healthy aging person recognizes are particularly present in the early morning hours. In this respect, we also expect a similar change in sleep and the subjectively perceived sleep quality. Where the immune system dominates in inflammatory diseases, chronic pain, chronic psychological stress, too much smoking, fear/anxiety, and chronic smoldering infections (see Part II of the book) must contribute to the increasing sleep problems in the elderly.

The interplay of the various unwanted energy expenditures has become known to us as a "double hit" or "multiple hit". Pain reduces sleep, reduced sleep stimulates more pain and more inflammation. Psychological stress, such as experienced

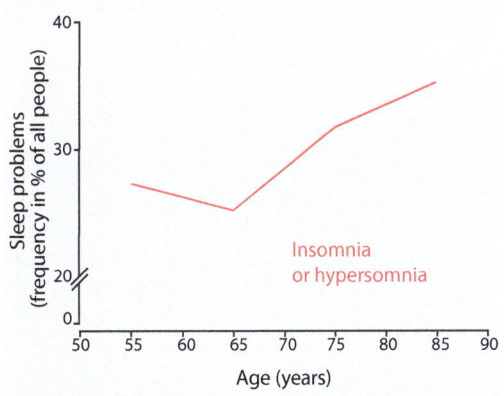

Increasing sleep problems in old age. As we age, subjectively reported sleep problems such as insomnia and hypersomnia steadily increase. Some people are prone to insomnia and others to hypersomnia.

■ **Fig. 10.4**   Increasing sleep problems in old age. (Data from Roberts et al. 2000)

with one's own illness, in the worry and care of a family member *(Care Giving)*, in loneliness and the like, changes the sleep quality and leads to more pain and higher inflammation. The higher inflammation stimulates more pain and sleep disorders, etc. In the end, the final result during aging is similar to chronic inflammation; there are higher unwanted energy expenditures. These unwanted energy expenditures prevent voluntary energy expenditures during the day through physical and mental activity, and this lack leads to the known problems of cardiovascular diseases, metabolic disorders, and declining mental activity.

References

Irwin MR, Straub RH, Smith MT (2023). Heat of the night: sleep disturbance activates inflammatory mechanisms and induces pain in rheumatoid arthritis. Nat Rev Rheumatol. 19:545–559

Roberts RE, Shema SJ, Kaplan GA, Strawbridge WJ (2000) Sleep complaints and depression in an aging cohort: A prospective perspective. Am J Psychiatry 157:81–88

Straub RH, Cutolo M (2007) Circadian rhythms in rheumatoid arthritis: implications for pathophysiology and therapeutic management. Arthritis Rheum 56:399–408

Wolkove N, Elkholy O, Baltzan M, Palayew M (2007) Sleep and aging: 1. Sleep disorders commonly found in older people. CMAJ 176:1299–1304

10

Loss of Appetite, Malnutrition, and Undernutrition

Contents

11.1   Appetite and Chronic Inflammation – 126

11.2   Anorexia of Aging – 127

References – 128

© The Author(s), under exclusive license to Springer-Verlag GmbH, DE, part of Springer Nature 2024
R. H. Straub, *Understanding Aging, Fatigue, and Inflammation*,
https://doi.org/10.1007/978-3-662-68904-2_11

11.1 Appetite and Chronic Inflammation

In ▶ Chap. 3 "Brain and Immune System—Two Competing Realms" it was discussed that a fight-or-flight response or an infection-dependent immune response leads to a loss of appetite. Loss of appetite is part of the *Sickness behavior*. When the two egoists, the brain or the immune system, are strongly activated, food intake is restricted or completely stopped. Searching for food under natural conditions cost a lot of extra energy, which can only take place without fight/flight or infection.

Here, we are reminded again of the study by the Japanese working group. Stone Age living male pygmies in Cameroon show during three consecutive days of hunting and searching for edible things, that less energy was taken in than was expended. This certainly cannot be a permanent state, and one must assume that there are better times for these Stone Age hunters in Cameroon. This simply tells us that under natural Stone Age conditions we have to expend a lot of energy for food search . An additional expenditure through fight/flight or infection must be avoided.

Therefore, the loss of appetite and the reduction of food intake in the context of *Sickness behavior* were conserved (positively selected) during evolution to save energy in an infection situation. However, if this reaction lasts too long, for example in a chronic inflammatory disease, problems such as malnutrition but also loss of muscle mass (▶ Chap. 12 "Muscle Loss") with simultaneous increase in relative fat mass (▶ Chap. 14 "Weight Changes") can be the result.

In rheumatoid arthritis, but also in many other chronic inflammatory diseases such as multiple sclerosis, food intake is reduced. Inevitably, the intake of other important factors such as fiber-rich diet, vitamins, iron, zinc, magnesium, calcium and others is reduced. Thus, loss of appetite also leads to the loss of valuable vital micronutrients and thus to malnutrition. In patients with chronic inflammatory diseases, food intake is lower the higher the inflammation parameters measured in the blood are.

A typical deficiency phenomenon is a significantly lower serum level of vitamin D, which is found to be reduced in almost all chronic inflammatory diseases. Vitamin D is an extremely important substance in bone and calcium metabolism, which serves the build-up of bone. Magnesium, calcium and phosphate are also essential factors in bone formation. Malnutrition promotes bone loss (▶ Chap. 13 "Bone Loss-Osteoporosis").

The reduced food intake in patients with rheumatoid arthritis is interestingly associated with the increased intake of unhealthy saturated fatty acids instead of healthy polyunsaturated fatty acids. The increased intake of saturated fatty acids with generally lower food intake has also been described in the chronic inflammatory disease of multiple sclerosis.

It is known that people under stressful life conditions react in a way that they rather look for high-calorie and energy-dense foods. These can then be sugar- and fat-rich snacks, which compensate for the energy loss of the active brain or immune system, but lack valuable micronutrients and have a high proportion of saturated fatty acids.

The group of Achim Peters from Lübeck was able to show that a short-term stress test over a few minutes led to a significantly increased consumption of high-calorie and energy-dense foods in the form of snacks. The intake of glucose in the snacks accounted for 25% of the daily consumption of the brain, although the increased brain performance only lasted a few minutes. If one looks at the amount of glucose and fat in the snacks, then the test persons showed an overcompensation.

This behavior is likely to have been positively selected for a state after a fight-or-flight response, but equally after the healing of an infection. We specifically seek out energy-dense and high-calorie foods, and this behavior is probably typical in situations with sudden energy expenditure. For short-term events, it makes sense because malnutrition and weight loss are to be expected. Weight loss and malnutrition need to be quickly corrected after the end of the acute event, and then we eat heartily. However, if the inflammation lasts too long, this program results in a mix of malnutrition and undernutrition.

11.2 Anorexia of Aging

The term "anorexia of aging" has been coined for similar nutritional problems of the aging, but otherwise healthy, person, i.e., loss of appetite in the aging person. Healthy older people are less hungry, are more satiated before and during meals, consume smaller meals, eat fewer high-calorie snacks between meals, and are quicker to feel full than young people before the age of 50. Healthy aging is also associated with the intake of a less variable and rather monotonous diet, as the sense of taste changes and, thus, the repeated intake of the same food is not disturbing. Normally, one avoids the repeated intake of the same food in order to achieve greater variability with a wider range of "good things". Finally, older people often suffer from malnutrition with a lack of protein-rich food.

If we look again at ◘ Fig. 8.2, we can see the striking reduction in total energy expenditure from the age of 50, as well as the loss of body mass without fat (fat-free mass: bones, muscles, and internal organs!) and the relative increase in fat mass. If you expend less energy from the age of 50, you must consequently also consume less energy. Between the ages of 20 and 80, daily energy intake decreases by up to 30%, so that by the age of 80, men consume 5,531 kJ (1,321 kcal) and women 2,633 kJ (629 kcal) less energy than at the age of 20. It is assumed that a large part of the reduced energy intake is due to a lower energy expenditure. However, in some people, energy intake is primarily lower than energy expenditure, which then leads to weight loss and inactivity.

Various studies on large populations have shown that people continue to gain weight until the age of 50-60, but that a continuous weight reduction is observed thereafter. On average, older Americans lose 4% of their weight per year from the age of 65. Due to weight loss and the higher mortality of overweight individuals before the age of 65, fewer and fewer people are overweight from the age of 65, and instead are more likely to be underweight.

But what are the reasons for decreased appetite?

The main reason cited is decreased physical and probably also mental activity, which is also expressed in ◘ Fig. 8.2 (there called AEE). This can be summarized by saying: "A higher degree of physical and mental inactivity leads to a lower need for food."

The following factors have often been mentioned:

- decreased sense of taste and therefore less interest in variable food,
- higher inflammatory activity,
- poorer gastrointestinal activity (smaller internal organs and altered movement patterns),
- lower serum levels of androgens such as testosterone or growth hormones (storage of energy-rich substrates in muscle and calcium, phosphate and magnesium in bone no longer takes place),
- higher levels of satiating hormones,
- stress-related phenomena such as loneliness (people eat more in company),
- depression and bereavement,
- dental problems,
- poverty in old age,
- problems with shopping or preparing food,
- chronic illness,
- frequent nausea or dizziness and the like.

The decreased physical activity results from the various additional unwanted energy expenditures present in old age, which were described in Part II of the book ("Energy Expenditures in the Spotlight"). With generally lower energy intake and additional food-consuming problems, there is a real energy shortage, which is most likely answered with reduced physical and mental activity. The reduced physical and mental activity is probably the leading cause of the "anorexia of aging" and the resulting complications such as cardiovascular diseases, metabolic diseases, etc.

11

References

Anderson L, Hadzibegovic DS, Moseley JM, Sellen DW (2014) Household food insecurity shows associations with food intake, social support utilization and dietary change among refugee adult caregivers resettled in the United States. Ecol Food Nutr 53:312–332

Chapman IM (2007) The anorexia of aging. Clin Geriatr Med 23:735–756

Hitze B, Hubold C, van DR, Schlichting K, Lehnert H, Entringer S, Peters A (2010) How the selfish brain organizes its supply and demand. Front Neuroenergetics 2:7–17

Rennie KL, Hughes J, Lang R, Jebb SA (2003) Nutritional management of rheumatoid arthritis: a review of the evidence. J Hum Nutr Diet 16:97–109

Shatenstein B, Kergoat MJ, Reid I (2007) Poor nutrient intakes during 1-year follow-up with community-dwelling older adults with early-stage Alzheimer dementia compared to cognitively intact matched controls. J Am Diet Assoc 107:2091–2099

Stamp LK, James MJ, Cleland LG (2005) Diet and rheumatoid arthritis: a review of the literature. Semin Arthritis Rheum 35:77–94

Straub RH (2015) The origin of chronic inflammatory systemic diseases and their sequelae. Academic, San Diego

Yamauchi T, Sato H (2000) Nutritional status, activity pattern, and dietary intake among the Baka hunter-gatherers in the village camps in cameroon. Afr Study Mongr 21:67–82

Muscle Loss

Contents

12.1   Muscle Loss and Chronic Inflammation – 130

12.2   Detour: Nutrition and Chronic Inflammation – 132

12.3   Muscle Mass Decreases with Age – 132

References – 135

The skeletal muscle stores large amounts of energy-rich proteins, which can be partially released when needed. In ► Chap. 1 on "Energy storage", we learned that the skeletal muscle stores about 50,000 kJ (12,000 kcal) of accessible energy, so that it can be used in an acute emergency. For a person who needs about 10,000 kJ (2388 kcal) per day, these protein reserves would be depleted after 5 days. In the case of absolute lack of food—for example during therapeutic fasting—the body draws the energy-rich substrates mainly from the muscle during the first 2 days. Only from the 3rd day onwards does the fat tissue take over the energy supply, the muscle is spared, and the fat tissue is broken down.

This fasting program has been maintained throughout our evolution (positively selected) to limit muscle breakdown as much as possible during energy-consuming times of crisis. The breakdown of muscle would be very unfavorable, as it would be associated with reduced physical activity and lack of movement. This would be followed by foraging problems, which would be difficult after advanced muscle breakdown. However, foraging or intake is essential after acute illness.

Put yourself in the position of our Stone Age ancestors, for we have inherited the relevant genes and mechanisms from them that were preserved during the process of evolution. In contrast, broken- down fat brings no functional disadvantages for mobility. On the contrary, one is significantly more mobile after the loss of fat reserves. In acute inflammatory situations with *Sickness behavior*, loss of appetite and fatigue, the muscle is therefore the first source of energy (for 2 days) and the fat tissue is second (from day 2 onward), although longer-lasting inflammatory situations are generally not allowed.

12.1 Muscle Loss and Chronic Inflammation

In chronic inflammatory disease, muscle loss is a glaring problem. Already in 1873, Dr. Lane from London described muscle loss in the context of long-lasting syphilis, which represents a chronic inflammatory situation. This was a time when syphilis was treated with mercury in the absence of penicillin, which ultimately helped little and somewhat prolonged the chronic phase with all its problems. The therapy with mercury was called the "therapeutic anchor of last resort", although it was very questionable as a treatment.

Muscle loss is also a typical problem in cancer diseases, when they are associated with a significantly increased energy expenditure (tumor growth needs energy). Muscle loss also occurs in cases of greatly increased mental activity in psychiatric and neurological diseases. Above, dementia was mentioned as well as Parkinson's or Huntington's etc.

Important investigations on the topic of muscle loss in the chronic inflammatory disease of rheumatoid arthritis come from Ronenn Roubenoff from the USA, who first described the phenomenon in 1990. At that time, he was working at Johns Hopkins University in Baltimore. The investigations were started because it was assumed that treatment with "cortisone" might lead to muscle loss. This side effect of this therapy was feared and muscle loss should be better defined. Since these patients were often treated in this way, the idea of muscle loss was obvious. This shows us, on the one hand, the importance of cortisone or the body's own cortisol for liberation of energy-rich substrates from the muscle (amino acids). On the other hand, it was the starting point for many important studies.

Roubenoff was later able to show that muscle loss in this disease did not depend solely on the administration of "cortisone" (also in many other diseases of a similar type). The chronic inflammatory disease caused muscle loss even when these medications were not administered. Just four years after the first description, he was able to show that muscle loss is primarily triggered by the cytokines released during high inflammation (TNF, interleukin-6 and interleukin-1). We had already learned about cytokines and the danger signals from dead cells as release factors of energy-rich substrates. It also becomes clear that this form of muscle loss was called inflammation-induced muscle loss.

The immune messenger substance TNF can have a very direct effect on the muscle and cause an immediate protein breakdown with the release of important amino acids. These amino acids can be used to produce glucose in the liver. The regenerated glucose is then passed on to the activated immune system, as glucose is the favorite food of the immune system. The chronic action of the cytokines also leads to a loss of muscle-building androgens and growth hormones. You will remember that sexual function and growth processes are shut down during inflammation because reproductive and courtship behavior or body growth and repair would consume too much energy. The shutdown of reproduction and growth was positively selected for short-term fight-or-flight reactions and acute infections in evolutionary history. However, it is used in a damaging way in chronic inflammatory disease.

The muscle loss is greatly exacerbated by muscular inactivity present in chronic inflammation. In ◘ Fig. 8.1, right column, it is shown how the additional energy expenditure by the activated immune system affects physical activity. Think of the *Sickness behavior*. Roubenoff showed that the energy expenditure through physical activity in patients with rheumatoid arthritis is about 1000 kJ (239 kcal) lower than in age-matched healthy individuals. This statement applies to patients who did not have severe inflammation because they were properly treated at the time and had not had a flare-up for more than 3 months. In an acute inflammatory flare-up, physical inactivity and thus immobility are likely to be much stronger.

It is also noticeable that muscle loss in patients with rheumatoid arthritis is not associated with a reduced body weight. One would expect this, as muscles weigh quite a lot. The muscle mass in patients with rheumatoid arthritis ranges from 7 to 35 kg in women and from 11 to 40 kg in men. So if a lot of muscle is lost, this should also result in a lower body weight. Interestingly, however, there is a reorganization of body composition, so that the missing muscle mass is replaced by an increased fat mass. This redistribution is unfavorable because it exacerbates physical inactivity and releases additional inflammatory factors from the enlarged adipose tissue.

Studies show that increasing strength or resistance training can significantly reduce or even reverse this muscle loss in patients with chronic inflammatory diseases. This applies equally to patients with cancer, osteoarthritis, chronic kidney diseases, chronic lung diseases, even heart failure or chronic HIV infection.

In the case of joint diseases, one always wonders whether the joints should be protected. Rest was also an element of the therapy recommendation three decades ago. Today we know that strength training in parallel to a causal anti-inflammatory therapy is beneficial. This strength training improves the long-term function of the affected limbs and also has beneficial effects on the rest of the body.

12.2 Detour: Nutrition and Chronic Inflammation

Here, a few points about nutrition in chronic inflammatory diseases such as rheumatoid arthritis should be mentioned. Between 35 and 75% of patients believe that they can control the disease through a certain dietary behavior. So it's not surprising that a lot is tried out here. Since these diseases were associated with allergic diseases 60 years ago, disease-causing food components were also thought of. It is therefore not surprising that food was selectively spared or selectively used.

It is also known that therapeutic fasting can inhibit inflammatory activity. This would not surprise us after everything said so far, because the withdrawal of energy-rich substrates also removes the energy for the active immune system. If the person concerned manages to lose weight starting from a too high body weight with generally less energy intake and expenditure, then the situation may be favorable insofar as the activated immune system would then also receive less energy. However, a well-controlled study of this possible therapeutic approach does not exist.

There is indeed literature that recommends a low-protein diet for these 'protein loss diseases' (muscle loss is a sign of protein loss). The author himself led such a debate in the family circle. The starting point of the discussion was a cautionary book that recommended a low-protein diet for inflammatory diseases. In these diseases, this is counterproductive, as the protein deficiency is in the foreground.

To this day, the therapy recommendations for these diseases are not based on large studies with modern design. Therefore, under no circumstances should a one-sided diet be followed, for example, without proteins. On the contrary, the diet should be balanced and variable and most closely resemble the so-called Mediterranean diet. In addition, it should be said that fish proteins are more favorable than proteins from red muscle meat, but even here there is no agreement because the large randomised controlled trials are simply missing.

12.3 Muscle Mass Decreases with Age

From the age of 30, we already lose 0.5–1% of muscle mass per year. By the age of 80, we have lost an incredible 30–40% of muscle mass compared to our 30th year of life. Approximately 10% of people aged 65 require assistance in daily life due to the effects of muscle loss. This percentage rises to over 50% for those who live beyond 85 years. It is estimated that about 1.5% of health system expenditures are caused by muscle loss. A reduction in the number of affected individuals by 10% would save about 1.1 billion US dollars in the USA. As the population in the developed countries of the Western world is getting older, the problems are steadily increasing.

Muscle loss in old age is associated with subsequent problems such as frailty, increasing immobility, fractures, bedriddenness, lower quality of life, and higher mortality.

Now let's turn to the causes of muscle loss during aging. In ◘ Fig. 8.2, the decreasing energy expenditure due to reduced physical activity in this stage of life was explained. Low physical activity and consequently loss of mobility are factors of the normal aging process. Inactivity, lack of androgens, and low growth hormone serum levels are central causes of muscle loss in old age. In this respect, the picture strikingly resembles chronic inflammatory diseases, in which these three factors also occur.

During aging, the loss of androgens is more attributable to the general decline in the performance of the hormone glands, whereas in chronic inflammatory diseases, high circulating inflammatory factors inhibit the function of the hormone-producing glands. Furthermore, food intake itself decreases during healthy aging. This results in a decline in protein-rich nutrition. Finally, neurological problems increase, so that the control of the muscles can become difficult. If additional unwanted energy expenditures are added (Part II of the book "Energy Expenditures in the Spotlight"), the decrease in physical activity is even greater, and the whole problem is intensified ("Double hit" or "Multiple hit"). ◘ Fig. 12.1 summarizes the causes again.

Muscle loss should be suspected if the following points are observed:

- frequent lying down (extreme: bedriddenness),
- rare walks,
- low walking speed (less than 8 m per 10 seconds or less than 2.9 km/hour),
- needing help when transitioning from a sitting position to a standing posture,
- preceding weight loss of more than 5% of body weight,
- significant loss of strength in the arms and hands,
- repeated falls,
- condition after hospital stay and
- other chronic diseases that make immobility more pronounced.

The essential therapeutic measure is **progressive muscle training** against external resistance, where the force to be overcome is slowly increased according to the individual's capabilities. The strength training can be supported by **endurance training** (e.g., home cycling).

The second measure is a balanced **diet**. Particular attention should be paid to adequate protein intake, as 40% of older people do not meet the minimum requirements of 0.8 grams of protein per kilogram of body weight. Thus, a protein intake of 1.5 grams per kilogram of body weight is recommended (about 200 g steak with beans, a cup of cottage cheese with fruits plus a large glass of milk), which corresponds to about 15–20% of the total energy intake.

Regarding the many other frequently mentioned dietary recommendations, there is little consensus. Thus, at most, a combined vitamin D and calcium supplementation is sensible in cases of confirmed bone loss. As for hormonal therapy with androgens (such as testosterone), one must be very cautious due to the side effects. Such therapy is only recommended for clearly proven, non-age-related deficiency of endogenous androgens. Unfortunately, there are no large-scale studies for most of the dietary and therapy suggestions. Lastly, it should be said that a combination of strength training and protein-appropriate nutrition inhibits muscle breakdown and promotes muscle growth.

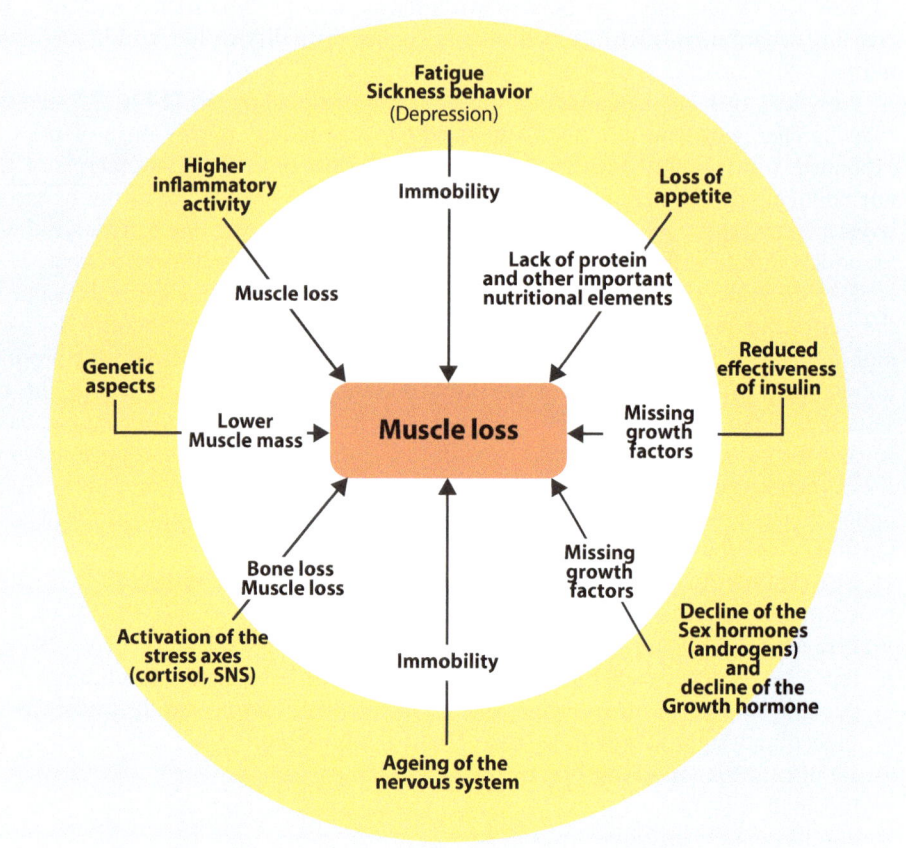

Causes of muscle wasting. The importance of insulin is discussed in chapter 15. SNS refers to the stress axis of the sympathetic nervous system, whose activity increases with age (see Chapter 17).

☑ **Fig. 12.1** Causes of muscle loss

It is clear that a person who is physically active during younger years is better off during aging, as they start from a different muscle mass at the onset of muscle loss. However, this only applies if they remain consistently active. In addition, this physically active individual has a different platform in terms of heart and lung function and the mental attitude towards physical activity. Therefore, the observable decrease in physical activity among today's young people, and hence the often too high body weight, will inevitably lead to more age-related muscle and bone problems.

12

References

Ali S, Garcia JM (2014) Sarcopenia, cachexia and aging: diagnosis, mechanisms and therapeutic options – a mini-review. Gerontology 60:294–305

Cooney JK, Law RJ, Matschke V, Lemmey AB, Moore JP, Ahmad Y, Jones JG, Maddison P, Thom JM (2011) Benefits of exercise in rheumatoid arthritis. J Aging Res: 681640

Rall LC, Rosen CJ, Dolnikowski G, Hartman WJ, Lundgren N, Abad LW, Dinarello CA, Roubenoff R (1996) Protein metabolism in rheumatoid arthritis and aging. Effects of muscle strength training and tumor necrosis factor alpha. Arthritis Rheum 39:1115–1124

Roubenoff R, Roubenoff RA, Cannon JG, Kehayias JJ, Zhuang H, wson-Hughes B, Dinarello CA, Rosenberg IH (1994) Rheumatoid cachexia: cytokine-driven hypermetabolism accompanying reduced body cell mass in chronic inflammation. J Clin Invest 93:2379–2386

Roubenoff R, Roubenoff RA, Ward LM, Stevens MB (1990) Catabolic effects of high-dose corticosteroids persist despite therapeutic benefit in rheumatoid arthritis. Am J Clin Nutr 52:1113–1117

Zinna EM, Yarasheski KE (2003) Exercise treatment to counteract protein wasting of chronic diseases. Curr Opin Clin Nutr Metab Care 6:87–93

Bone Loss—Osteoporosis

Contents

13.1   Bone Loss and Chronic Inflammation – 138

13.2   Bone Loss in Old Age – 140

References – 141

▶ Chapter 1 among other things, showed the regulation of energy storage in the human body. There, in ◙ Fig. 1.8 besides the typical storage places for glucose, fatty acids, and amino acids—namely adipose tissue, muscle tissue, and liver—the bone was also mentioned. The bone is the largest storage for calcium, phosphate, and magnesium. These chemical elements are necessary for many cell functions, which is why a supply must be available.

During our evolutionary history, our ancestors left the sea for land about 350 million years ago. In the sea, there was always enough calcium, magnesium and phosphate, as these elements are present in high quantities in seawater. Especially during the transition to land, a storage of these special chemical elements was necessary because one was no longer constantly surrounded by seawater. The bone is an incredibly large reservoir for calcium, phosphate, and magnesium.

We owe important studies on bone loss—osteoporosis—to the Innsbruck doctor Gustav A. Pommer, born in 1851, who focused his interest on the tissue examination of the bone. Pommer recognized the thinning of the bone in people with increasing age. Bone metabolism is still a domain of Austrian research today.

Nowadays, the quality of the bone is examined with bone density measurements. This examination is usually carried out at several points of the skeleton. It became clear that bone loss is typical for chronic inflammatory diseases, but also characteristic during aging.

13.1 Bone Loss and Chronic Inflammation

In chronic inflammatory disease, bone loss, similar to muscle loss, is a serious problem. Similar to muscle loss, the causative elements of bone thinning are diverse.

First and foremost, the inadequate intake of food should be mentioned here, which we have encountered in chronic inflammatory disease, but also during aging. Consequently, the intake of other important factors such as fiber-rich diet, vitamins, iron, zinc, magnesium, calcium, and others is reduced. Thus, the inflammation-related loss of appetite also leads to the loss of valuable vital micronutrients and thus to relative malnutrition.

A typical deficiency phenomenon is a significantly lower serum level of biologically active vitamin D, which was discussed in ▶ Chap. 11 as a result of malnutrition (it is found in fatty fish like herring, offal, eggs, and to a limited extent also in dairy products). Vitamin D is an important substance in bone metabolism, which serves the build-up of the bone. Magnesium, calcium, and phosphate are also essential factors in bone formation. The loss of appetite and malnutrition promote bone loss due to a lack of essential factors.

Secondly, the high activity of the immune system in chronic inflammatory disease should be mentioned. It stimulates firstly the *Sickness behavior* and thus leads to a lack of physical activity. However, a lack of physical activity is an important factor for bone loss. Thus, one study showed that about 35% of bone loss was due to a lack of physical activity. Another study on accident victims shows the correlation between lack of movement and an increase in calcium excretion in the urine, which is considered an indirect measure of bone degradation. The lack of movement led to a significant increase in calcium excretion after just 4 weeks. While at the beginning of the injury treatment 0% had an increased calcium level in the urine, after 4 weeks it was 64% in the accident victims. This shows the enormous bone degradation during the first period of lack of movement.

Then, we should be reminded of muscle loss again, because muscle loss promotes bone loss due to increasing lack of movement. As we have seen, muscle loss in chronic inflammation is a program to release energy-rich substrates from the muscle and play them to the selfish immune system (glucogenic amino acids).

Normally, bone metabolism is regulated by hormones that control both the growth and breakdown in such a way that a balance is maintained. In healthy individuals, hormones are the essential control elements of bone metabolism (parathyroid hormone, androgens, estrogens, vitamin D, growth hormone). The high activity of the immune system in chronic inflammatory disease fundamentally changes this situation, as the importance of hormones recedes into the background. Important cytokines such as TNF, interleukin-6 and interleukin-1, but also immune cells, can very directly activate bone breakdown. This special importance of the activated immune system can only be understood if one takes into account evolutionary medicine.

Under acute infection conditions for a maximum of 2–3 weeks with insufficient food intake during *Sickness behavior*, the release of calcium, phosphate, and magnesium is important to compensate for the food-related deficiency within these 2–3 weeks. The selfish immune system therefore releases the necessary factors that very directly promote bone breakdown. So, no one—not even the hormone glands—is asked whether this is a sensible approach of the selfish immune system. All is well if it only lasts a short time. In chronic inflammatory diseases, this program preserved in our evolutionary history is constantly used, so that bone loss regularly occurs.

In third place is the inflammation-related decrease in androgen levels. Androgens are important growth factors for muscles and bones, which is why their loss is disadvantageous. This issue is explained in detail in ▶ Chap. 16.

In fourth place, we have learned that the stress axes—the hypothalamus-pituitary-adrenal axis and especially the sympathetic nervous system—are activated during inflammation. The hormones of these two stress axes—both cortisol and adrenaline/noradrenaline—break down bone. Since the activity of the sympathetic nervous system is particularly increased in chronic inflammatory disease, adrenaline and noradrenaline can contribute to bone loss.

If these various pathways are used during acute inflammation, they are useful because they supply the body with calcium, phosphate, and magnesium. However, with long-term use of this program in the context of a chronic inflammatory disease, bone loss of destructive proportions occurs.

Typically, a higher calcium intake plus vitamin D is therapeutically recommended. But first and foremost is the medicinal suppression of inflammatory activity, as most problems originate from here (◘ Fig. 13.1). Sometimes, bone loss in chronic inflammatory diseases can be so severe that highly effective inhibitors of bone-degrading cells must be used (bisphosphonates, antibodies against the bone-degrading protein RANKL [Denosumab]).

The administration of androgens has been studied in chronic inflammatory diseases, and there were indications of an improvement in the bone situation, but this therapy did not find its way into clinical practice, although especially men with low androgen levels would benefit.

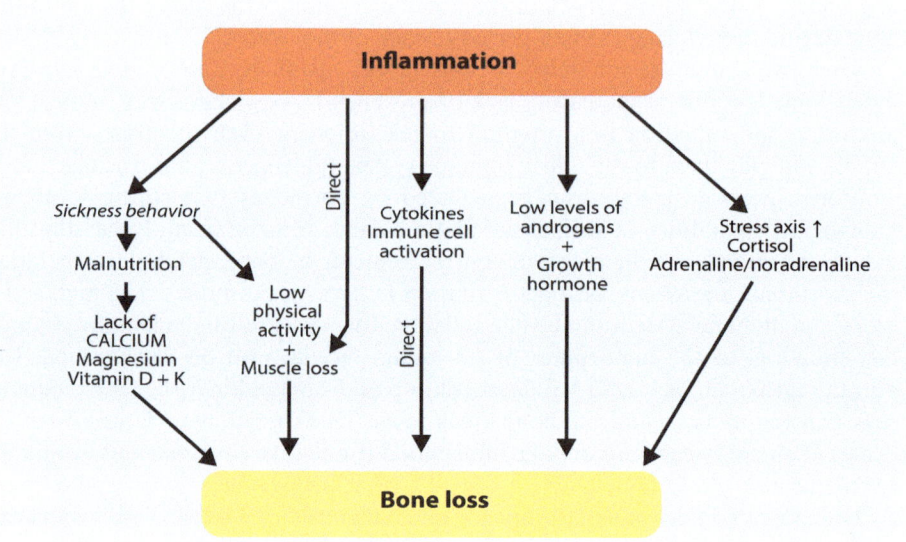

■ **Fig. 13.1**   Causes of inflammation-related bone loss

Probably, the above-mentioned highly effective inhibitors of bone breakdown are so dominantly marketed that these other options are not in the focus of interest. In addition, muscle training and physical activity are important to minimize bone loss caused by lack of movement.

13.2 Bone Loss in Old Age

13

We learned that inflammation during aging is somewhat increased, but cannot be equated with chronic inflammatory diseases. Therefore, in old age, some other factors must be responsible for bone loss.

First and foremost, loss of appetite and malnutrition, which was called "anorexia of aging", should be mentioned. Thus, in old age there is malnutrition for non-inflammatory reasons, which leads to reduced intake of essential bone-growth factors (calcium, magnesium, vitamin D, vitamin K). In addition, sun exposure, which is needed for the production of the body's own biologically active vitamin D, is lower in old age. Many elderly people no longer want to show off their bodies, which contributes to a lack of sun exposure.

Secondly, the reduced physical activity of aging people is important. For the reasons mentioned in Book Part II, such as smoldering inflammation, chronic pain, various forms of psychological stress, fears, caring for family members, sleep problems, and the like, there is an increasing reduction in physical activity, which promotes muscle and bone loss.

Thirdly, the loss of androgens and estrogens in old age is evident. Especially women experience a significant increase in bone loss after menopause. In fact, men are also affected due to the increase of hormone loss, but men generally start from a higher initial value of bone and muscle mass, so the problem shows up less or later.

Fourthly, the increase in the activity of the stress axes adds to the problem, because in relation to the other hormones—especially the sex hormones—cortisol does not decrease during aging, and hormones of the sympathetic nervous system even increase (noradrenaline and adrenaline). This imbalance promotes bone degradation.

In fact, large studies with inhibitors of the sympathetic nervous system (also called β-blockers, which are prescribed for high blood pressure or heart failure) show that the intake of these β-blockers is associated with a reduced bone fracture rate. Since bone fracture is a sign of bone loss, the β-blocker-induced reduction in the number of bone fractures is an indication of the unfavorable effects of the sympathetic nervous system on the bone.

Thus, elderly people are affected by bone loss for slightly different reasons than younger people with chronic inflammation, but in principle very similar mechanisms as in chronic inflammatory disease play the decisive role.

Physical activity is the decisive factor, as voluntarily increased activity leads to increased food intake and to a stronger build-up of muscle and bone. Moderate physical activity is also associated with better sleep, fewer psychological stress phenomena, less pain, for example in the context of arthritis, and less inflammation.

References

Straub RH, Cutolo M, Pacifici M (2015) Evolutionary medicine and bone loss in chronic inflammatory diseases – a theory of inflammation-related osteopenia. Semin Arthritis Rheum 45:220–228

van Marken Lichtenbelt WD, Heidendal GA, Westerterp KR (1997) Energy expenditure and physical activity in relation to bone mineral density in women with anorexia nervosa. Eur J Clin Nutr 51:826–830

Yusuf MB, Ikem IC, Oginni LM, Akinyoola AL, Badmus TA, Idowu AA, Orimolade AE (2013) Comparison of serum and urinary calcium profile of immobilized and ambulant trauma patients. Bone 57:361–366

Weight Changes (Increase and Decrease)

Contents

14.1   Weight and Chronic Inflammation – 144

14.2   Weight During Aging – 144
14.2.1   Obesity is on the Rise – 145
14.2.2   Weight Gain and Evolutionary Medicine – 147
14.2.3   Overcompensation Leads to Weight Gain – 148
14.2.4   Ignorance Leads to Weight Gain – 150
14.2.5   Weight Gain: Physical Activity – 150
14.2.6   Weight Gain or Weight Loss in Stressful Life
          Circumstances – 152

References – 154

© The Author(s), under exclusive license to Springer-Verlag GmbH, DE, part of Springer Nature 2024
R. H. Straub, *Understanding Aging, Fatigue, and Inflammation*,
https://doi.org/10.1007/978-3-662-68904-2_14

14.1 Weight and Chronic Inflammation

In chronic inflammatory diseases, we have come to know a highly to higher active immune system that consumes a lot of energy. It has been shown that energy expenditure can be on the order of 2100 kJ (500 kcal) per day. So it is not surprising that this higher energy expenditure hardly leads to weight gain, but rather must lead to weight loss.

In fact, patients with various chronic inflammatory diseases are not obese, but usually of normal weight. Especially children show typical growth disorders and a lower age-related body weight under these conditions.

A high to normal or overweight body mass is nowadays often present thanks to good anti-inflammatory therapy, which significantly reduces the energy expenditure of the immune system. In times without anti-inflammatory drugs, weight loss was the rule, and this phenomenon was sometimes labeled "emaciation".

It is also interesting that patients with chronic inflammatory diseases have a milder form of the disease and fewer disease consequences if they have a high body weight. This was called a paradox because normally people with high body weight are more likely to suffer from secondary diseases such as cardiovascular diseases—heart attack and stroke—or metabolic diseases—diabetes in old age—or high blood pressure. But with chronic inflammatory diseases, it is the other way around: there, those patients with high body weight are protected relative to all others with the same disease because they probably have a milder course of the disease, in which less energy is needed by the immune system. The immune system is therefore less active, the inflammation is less pronounced, and since the inflammation can already lead to secondary diseases, there are fewer of them in the presence of a milder disease.

The possible weight loss due to loss of appetite, malnutrition, muscle loss, and bone loss could already be anticipated. The reduction of muscle and bone mass must lead to lower body weight in chronic inflammatory disease, but also in old age. It was also shown that in well-treated chronic inflammatory diseases and during normal healthy aging, a redistribution from fat-free mass to fat-rich mass takes place. This redistribution is unfavorable because the willingness to physical activity dwindles with lower muscle mass in relation to high fat mass. In addition, increased fat mass is associated with slightly higher inflammatory activity because the adipose tissue produces inflammatory factors such as interleukin-6 itself.

In summary, it can be said that chronic inflammatory diseases rarely go hand in hand with obesity, but rather with normal weight or at most in these times with good therapies with moderate overweight.

14.2 Weight During Aging

During the aging process, we go through an important transition around the age of 50, because from then on, less and less total energy is consumed and expended. Furthermore, the energy expenditure for physical activities steadily decreases (◘ Fig. 8.2). There is an increasing weight loss with malnutrition, muscle loss, shrinkage of internal organs, and bone loss, which can be observed particularly from the age of 65.

Nevertheless, many people are getting heavier, and some experience this especially in the years up to the age of 65. The consideration of weight gain must refer to the entire lifetime, as often the platform for weight development up to the age of 65 is determined already in the womb and in childhood.

Before discussing the individual aspects of weight gain, we take stock.

14.2.1 Obesity is on the Rise

When the so-called *Body Mass Index* (BMI = weight in "kg" divided by height in "m" squared) is equal to or greater than 30 kg/m², it is referred to as obesity.

Body Mass Index (BMI)
BMI = Body weight (kg)/Body length squared (m²)
- Underweight: BMI <18.5
- Normal weight: BMI ≥18.5–25
- Overweight: BMI >25–29.99
- Obesity: BMI ≥30

Obesity is a significant issue in the modern world (◘ Fig. 14.1). One is considered overweight with a BMI between 25 and less than 30 kg/m² and normal weight between 18.5 and less than 25 kg/m². The Body Mass Index is only partially useful, as it does not provide information about body composition (i.e., lean muscle versus fat tissue).

Obesity or fatness is unfortunately on the rise. In 1973, only 14.0% of Americans were obese, today it is 40%. The increase affects all Western countries more or less strongly. The problems of obesity are manifold, and it is quite clear that obesity is associated with a higher risk of subsequent diseases such as cardiovascular diseases, such as heart attack and stroke, type 2 diabetes, hypertension, joint diseases, depression, cancer, etc. A mild inflammatory situation arises in the adipose tissue, which is held responsible for these many subsequent diseases.

One could rightly ask why there can be inflammation—yes, chronic inflammation—in adipose tissue. There is currently no comprehensive answer to this, but it should be said right away that this inflammation is of a mild nature and cannot be equated with that in chronic inflammatory diseases such as rheumatoid arthritis. Consider again ◘ Fig. 4.2. It is shown there that obesity is associated with a blood level of 5.0 pg/ml interleukin-6 (as high as in a caregiver of an Alzheimer's patient). This is chronic in obesity, but by no means very energy-consuming (this shows ◘ Fig. 4.3).

With this interleukin-6 level, it can be seen that energy expenditure would not even increase by 250 kJ (60 kcal) per day. To put it bluntly: "The energy expenditure due to obesity-related inflammation is not sufficient to reverse obesity through this energy expenditure." This is different in chronic inflammatory diseases, where there are almost no obese people. There, the energy expenditure is high enough that

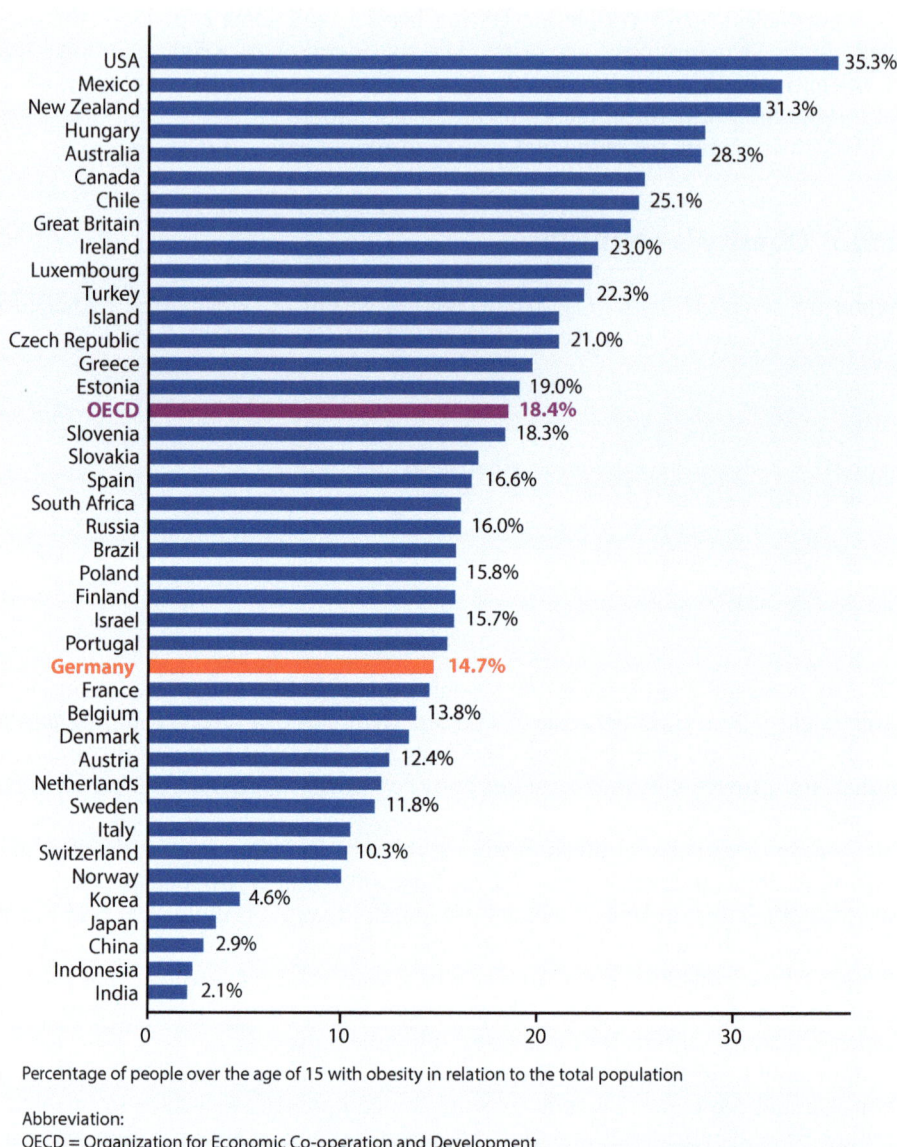

Percentage of people over the age of 15 with obesity in relation to the total population

Abbreviation:
OECD = Organization for Economic Co-operation and Development
Data from the current OECD Obesity Update 2014, available at the following URL:
http://www.oecd.org/health/obesity-update.htm

Fig. 14.1 Percentage of people over the age of 15 with obesity. (Data from the Organisation for Economic Co-operation and Development—OECD 2014)

little reserves can be stored. The immune system constantly consumes too much (especially without adequate therapy).

The preceding considerations also make it clear that obesity occurs when more energy is taken in and stored than is expended through various activities. This

14

simple balance calculation is well known, and that's exactly where the crux of the matter lies.

14.2.2 Weight Gain and Evolutionary Medicine

Basically, it is very advantageous if we have enough reserves, because food shortages and energy-consuming activities in fight/flight and infections have always been an issue. Therefore, it can be assumed that some genes and the mechanisms dependent on them were preserved (positively selected) in the evolutionary process to build up these stores. Indeed, such genes have been found in recent years. However, the disappointment was great, as the genetic traits found so far could not explain even 10% of the genetic causes of obesity. So what is it then?

A fascinating finding came from population-based studies by the working group around David Barker (1938–2013), who taught clinical epidemiology in Southampton, UK. Barker discovered the important correlation between food shortages during development in the womb (e.g., maternal hunger) and the later development of obesity in the child. The more and larger the shortages in energy supply were, the more obese children became at a young age before puberty.

It must be assumed that the shortages in energy supply set important switches and adjust control variables that later lead to rapid weight gain. Since this situation only becomes relevant in the living fetus after the occurrence of a shortage, it is not written in the genes of the fetus from the beginning. This flexibility or plasticity serves to adapt to environmental conditions (epigenetic causes).

Assuming that these shortages in the fetus stimulate a signal for energy deficiency, then the fetus seems to prepare for a lean time (low energy) after birth. After birth, the child tries to gain weight quickly to better meet the demands. The child builds up energy stores. This phenomenon has been confirmed in humans, but also in many different animal species. This cause of the later developing obesity explains much more comprehensively why obesity can occur later in life. Children of malnourished mothers experience an energy shortage and develop the described phenomenon.

Barker demonstrated this in people who were born between 1911 and 1930 in Hertfordshire, England. Children of mothers with obesity probably already experience a similar energy shortage in the womb because the mother competes for the energy-rich substrates. This could well explain the familial accumulation of obesity, without special genetic traits having to play a role.

Since the phenomenon is significant both in animals such as rats and mice, which had the last common ancestor to humans about 65 million years ago, and in humans themselves, it was deeply rooted in our common ancestor and is deeply rooted in today's rats and mice and in humans. Here, obesity is established before puberty, so it can be assumed that this plastic phenomenon in the evolutionary history of animals and humans could not have been a disadvantage. On the contrary, there must have been an evolutionary advantage. From this evolutionary medical perspective, the predisposition to obesity would basically be favorable. But what is the problem then?

In the times of the Stone Age lifestyle of humans, food surplus was rare, and therefore obesity was rare. It was only reserved for the powerful and privileged, and it was a beauty ideal or something to strive for, as the Venus of Willendorf still teaches us today. This Venus figure was found in 1908 in Willendorf in the Wachau (Austria). It is a female, naked, very obese female figure made of limestone, which can be admired today in the Vienna Museum of Natural History.

Even in our more recent history, obesity was only an issue for the rich and great, who were then also plagued by gout and cardiovascular diseases. Because only those who can supply enough energy over a longer period of time achieve the format of the Venus of Willendorf. The Barker phenomenon probably rarely came into long-term use in our evolutionary history. However, it must have been important as a storage mechanism, as we can still observe this phenomenon today—more than ever. The platform for the Barker phenomenon was not abolished in evolutionary history to disappear, but positively selected to stay.

With these insights, it is easy to understand why one can become obese today. But why does this happen, even though it is not advantageous today?

14.2.3 Overcompensation Leads to Weight Gain

There are many causes for obesity, and it would probably exceed the scope of this book if all causes were to be listed in detail. One thing is certain, if you become obese, you have taken in and stored more energy than you have expended and lost.

The study by Achim Peters from Lübeck was introduced earlier. To remind you, it is briefly summarized again. In an acute psychological stress test over 15 minutes, this study showed an overcompensation of voluntary energy intake after the test in the form of highly tasty energy-dense snacks from an otherwise rich buffet. Overcompensation means that too many energy-rich substrates were taken in relation to the test-related energy expenditure. The ten-minute test led to a stress-related increase in intake of 26% of the energy needed daily by the brain, which corresponds to about 571 kJ (137 kcal). Obviously, the body overcompensated because it wanted to reward itself. Peters says: "The brain is selfish regarding energy desires."

Overcompensation also occurs under other conditions that people find stressful. For example, in poorer families, the food supply can sometimes be unstable, leading to food scarcity. However, this lack of food does not lead to a lower energy intake, as one would actually expect. In better times, high-calorie and energy-dense snacks are consumed in large quantities. Women and children are particularly affected by this. So, in better times, there is overcompensation, with sweets and sweet juices being preferred. Sweet foods are perceived as a reward.

Another form of chronic stress is chronic insomnia or shift-related sleep disorders, which lead to a higher energy expenditure (▶ Chap. 7 "Sleep disorders and circadian symptoms"). In the case of chronic insomnia and lack of muscle relaxation, there is an increased appetite, which can be explained by the increased need for energy. However, if overcompensation were to occur here, as described above in the psychological stress test from Lübeck, the energy intake could be significantly higher than the energy expenditure caused by lack of sleep. The consequence would be unwanted weight gain.

Since sleep disorders actually lead to an increase in diabetes and obesity, there is much to suggest overcompensation and other disturbances of the energy balance. A recent study showed that energy intake undoubtedly exceeds the increased energy

14

expenditure. This increased energy intake occurs particularly late at night, and these correlations have now been confirmed by other authors. Again, high-calorie foods with a high sugar and fat content, specifically the unfavorable saturated fatty acids, are preferred. They are perceived as a reward or compensation for lack of sleep.

Furthermore, stressed people often drink too much alcohol to calm down and sleep better. The effect on falling asleep and staying asleep alone is a well-known reason for chronic alcohol abuse. In this situation, large amounts of energy are consumed (a bottle of white wine contains about 2575 kJ [615 kcal], a bottle of beer about 900 kJ [215 kcal]).

However, since alcohol has an aftereffect the next day and makes you tired, it leads to a reduced energy expenditure with decreased physical activity. In addition, alcohol stimulates the appetite, so high-calorie snacks are often consumed alongside alcohol intake. Although this is not well studied, the stress that triggers it is likely to consume less energy than is later supplied by alcohol. Such reward behavior then leads to overcompensation especially in men (see below, ◘ Table 14.1). In severe alcoholism, however, weight loss is often observed, as for example the conversion to fatty acids in the diseased liver and the storage of fatty acids in the adipose tissue increasingly function poorly.

Long-term police work with a high stress potential very often leads to overweight and obesity. These individuals were also more often chronically ill and showed signs of depression and overwork more frequently. And children are particularly at risk when the home is disharmonious, when there are socioeconomic

◘ **Table 14.1** Characteristics of chronically stressed individuals who gain or lose weight

40% Weight gain	40% Weight loss
*Are at the upper end of normal weight or above at the beginning of the observation	Are normal weight or underweight at the beginning of the observation
Lower level of education	Higher level of education
Little social support at work	Good social support at work
Low intake of vegetables and fruits	High intake of vegetables
Low intake of fiber-rich food	High proportion of fiber-rich food
Many high-calorie snacks (sugar, fat)	Few high-calorie snacks (sugar, fat)
More alcohol (in men)	No alcohol (in men)
Low physical activity	High physical activity (2 hours of intense training per week)
Low sense of satisfaction (in women)	High degree of openness (in men)
Often neurotic behavior (in women)	
Low activation of stress axes in response to stress ('cool' types)	High activation of stress axes in response to stress ('hectic' types)
Low activation of stress axes in response to repeated stress of the same type	High activation of stress axes in response to repeated stress of the same type

* These individuals have probably already shown the pattern of weight gain before the start of the observation

problems, when parents pass on frustration, when parental support is lacking, when a negative worldview is developed, when there are large emotional needs, and when a generally insecure life situation must be assumed. Such children often have low self-esteem, negative emotions, powerlessness, depression, anxiety, feelings of insecurity, and problems with stressful life situations. This psycho-emotional overload often leads to overcompensatory food intake of high-calorie and energy-dense snacks, which is perceived as an immediate reward.

However, it should be noted at this point that not all people gain weight under stressful life circumstances. Studies on large population groups show that 40% gain weight, 40% lose weight, and 20% remain about the same. So when we talk about obesity in stressful life circumstances, this only applies to 40% of people. The reason for weight loss will be explained in the last section of this chapter.

14.2.4 Ignorance Leads to Weight Gain

Another cause of obesity is ignorance of the amount of food or energy consumed. Imagine being asked one day before going to sleep what foods you have consumed. In your answer, you neglect the food with high-calorie snacks. This is what is meant by ignorance.

If a person does not admit to themselves the amount of energy consumed or does not correctly estimate it based on a given target value, there is a risk of consuming too much energy. Several studies have shown that people did not correctly estimate the amount of energy when
- they had a high body weight,
- they had a higher fat mass,
- the perceived stress load was high, and
- they were more likely to be male.

It also turned out that these people consumed less calcium, fiber-rich diet, iron, vitamin B1/B6, and ate fewer fruits and vegetables.

Thus, the overweight consumed 1675 kJ (400 kcal) and the normal weight 1130 kJ (270 kcal) more energy per day than they had indicated in the food questionnaires. Even the normal weight were somewhat ignorant, but the overweight were more ignorant. This difference can lead to increasing body weight over the years. Basically, this is a cycle of overcompensation, ignorance, high fat mass/low muscle mass, and reduced physical activity.

14.2.5 Weight Gain: Physical Activity

Compared to our closest relatives, the great apes, taking into account body size and body weight, we have a significantly higher daily turnover of about 2512 kJ (600 kcal). Therefore, we also consume more energy, and the basal metabolic rate, which was mentioned in ▢ Fig. 8.1, is also significantly higher. The anthropologist Herman Pontzer from New York and his colleagues recently compiled these findings in the scientific journal *Nature*. Pontzer found that this additional energy expenditure is largely due to a more active brain. An active selfish brain, according to the considerations from Part I of the book, is also strongly associated with higher physical and mental activity, unless it is prevented by a selfish immune system.

If we expend more energy than the great apes, then we must also be careful not to run into energy shortages. We probably do this by being able to store energy in adipose tissue better than the great apes. This would mean that in the 6–7 million years that separate us from a common ancestor of today's great apes, better fat storage was positively selected in human evolution.[1]

In 2012, Pontzer made another important discovery after observing the Hadza, a Stone Age people living near Lake Eyazi in Tanzania. He found that among these hunters and gatherers, the total energy expenditure per day, taking into account body size and body weight, is very similar to that of people living in the Western world. This is very surprising, and it can be concluded that the total energy expenditure is a feature independent of culture and living conditions.

This consideration is linked to another insight. As a rule, energy expenditure matches energy intake, as otherwise we would constantly lose or gain weight. Since the Hazda and Western-living humans expend the same total amount of energy, they must also consume a similar amount of energy. This should also be a feature independent of culture in normal-weight individuals.

However, Pontzer also found that the physical activity of the Stone Age-living Hazda is significantly greater compared to people of the affluent society, and the basal metabolic rate (BMR in ◘ Fig. 8.1) for the basic supply of organs is significantly smaller. So, the Western-living human has a high energy expenditure for the basic supply of organs. The high basal metabolic rate, however, does not mean energy expenditure through physical movement (BMR in ◘ Fig. 8.1). In addition, the basal metabolic rate of the Western-living human as measured in this way also includes a higher energy expenditure by the immune system (e.g., in adipose tissue), which cannot be separately represented and investigated with the common measurement methods.

Therefore, the Western-living human does not consume more energy than the Hazda (taking into account body dimensions), but he expends it for the basal supply of organs including the immune system and not for physical activity. In summary, the contemporary living in the Western world moves less, but still consumes a lot of energy and can store this energy better than any great ape, especially in adipose tissue.

We spoke of energy shortages, which is why there is a higher fat storage in us compared to the great apes. Considering the desired and the additional unwanted energy expenditures, the problem of the energy shortage is exacerbated. The unwanted energy expenditures lead to reduced physical activity and reward behavior (► Chap. 8), and this increasingly worsens the overall situation. On this basis, a vicious cycle can arise, which is associated with overcompensation and weight gain. This vicious cycle is shown in ◘ Fig. 14.2.

---

1 Another consideration: Since great apes living under natural conditions in the tropics, compared to humans living in colder areas, need less energy to maintain body temperature, it is understandable that humans, unlike great apes, conserved (positively selected) mechanisms during the course of evolutionary history that brought about higher energy storage. Yet another consideration: Perhaps the Barker phenomenon is also less in great apes because they live in food-rich areas and therefore experience fewer fetal energy shortages.

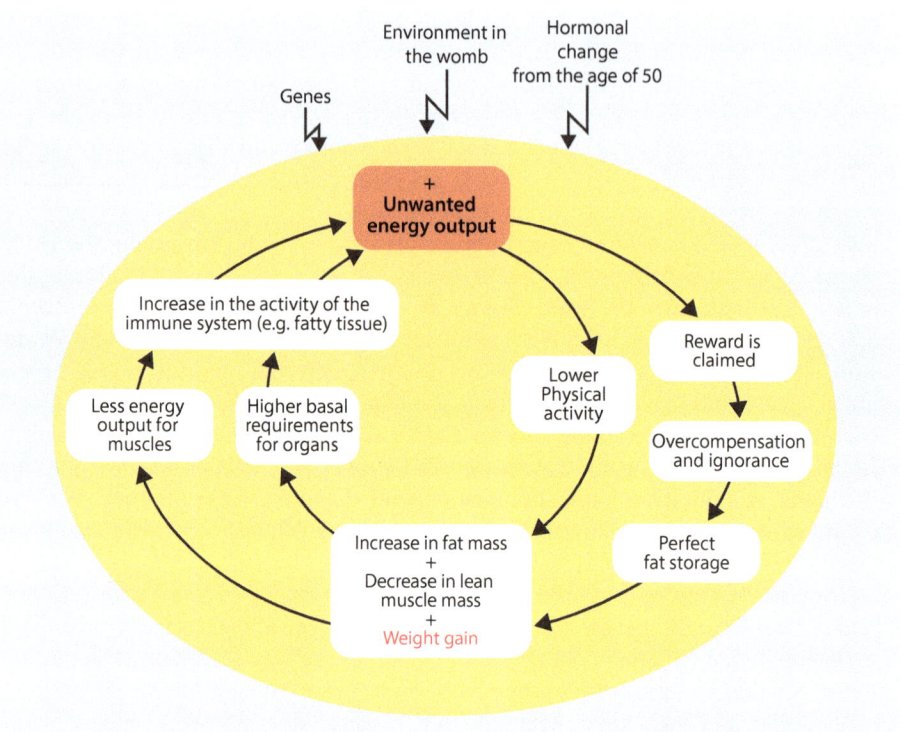

Vicious cycle of weight gain. Unwanted energy expenditure (inflammation, smoldering inflammation, pain, psychological stress [e.g. care giving or dementia], anxiety, sleep problems, too much smoking, etc.) leads to energy deprivation, reduced physical activity and reward behaviors. It is overcompensated with less valuable foods (high-calorie snacks with sugar and saturated fatty acids or alcohol), the overcompensation is ignored and energy-rich substrates are perfectly stored in fatty tissue. The fat mass increases steadily, the muscle mass decreases steadily, there is a higher basic requirement of the organs and a lower energy expenditure by the muscles. The increase in adipose tissue causes an increase in the activity of the immune system, and together with unwanted energy expenditure of other kinds, the process is constantly exacerbated. The consequences are weight gain with higher fat mass and a decrease in fat-free mass. This system (in yellow) is influenced by the general conditions, the genes, the situation in the womb (Barker phenomenon!) and the forced change of the hormone glands during the menopause (woman) and andropause (man) (lightning symbols above).

14

◘ **Fig. 14.2**   Vicious cycle of weight gain

14.2.6 Weight Gain or Weight Loss in Stressful Life Circumstances

Only 40% of people gain weight under stressful life events of various kinds. Overall, 40% lose weight under these circumstances and 20% remain constant. Those with constant weight are to be envied because they seem to do everything right during the stressful time. They are probably the ones with the golden mean.

An enlightening study comes from England, conducted on students of the *University College of London* in their first year after starting their studies. First-year students experienced the demands as a chronically stressful event. In 80% the eating behavior changed, with 42% reporting reduced and 38% increased food intake. Stressed students ate more high-calorie snacks, whereas the intake of fruits, vegetables, meat, and fish decreased. Further studies with individuals exposed to various forms of psychological stress found similar numbers regarding weight gain and loss. Typical characteristics of the two groups were summarized in ◘ Table 14.1.

It is obvious that the "losers" have a higher stress axis activity and a higher physical activity than the "gainers". We have learned that high stress axis activity is associated with the breakdown of energy-rich substrates. The losers are the more active people, and they also eat healthier. Perhaps it has something to do with the level of education, as they may have sought more information on proper health behavior. In any case, the level of education is higher among the losers than among the gainers.

If you take another form of physical stress for this consideration, for example, physical illness, then you might find in a similar way that physical activity is key to understanding the two weight types. In ▶ Chap. 6 "Psychological Stress and Energy" it was already explained that physical illness means not only physical stress but also psychological stress. Therefore, the conditions with weight gain and loss might be similar.

Klaas Westerterp is a professor of human energy regulation at the University of Maastricht in the Netherlands. He examined patients with chronic obstructive pulmonary disease. Chronic obstructive pulmonary disease is known, for example, in asthmatics and chronic smokers, in whom the small airways narrow, partly clog with mucus, and have a thicker wall. In crisis situations—e.g., inflammation and infection of the airways—the patient experiences shortness of breath. In chronic situations, there is increasing narrowing and wall thickening. Good therapy reduces the problem. In this group of patients, Westerterp's working group found losers and gainers. It should be said right away that the inflammation constellation was somewhat higher, but by no means as high as in chronic inflammatory diseases. So it must be something else!

Westerterp was able to determine in these patients that they had a higher total energy expenditure compared to healthy individuals. If the total energy expenditure was broken down into the basal metabolic rate and the energy expenditure caused by physical activity as in ◘ Fig. 8.1, these patients showed a relatively high physical activity when they were seriously ill. The energy expenditure for the immune system was not higher than in healthy people. But why is there a higher physical activity in these patients?

Shortness of breath is no fun, and the affected person is driven to constantly create favorable conditions for improved breathing. This can be done, for example, by raising the upper body or by high breathing frequency. Increased energy expenditures also result from sleep problems. The patients wake up at night, raise their upper body steeply, and breathe in and out with a lot of effort. This happens especially in the early morning hours, where even the healthy person produces more obstructive mucus. This is also a circadian symptom with a peak in the early morning hours. The repeated application of therapeutic procedures against chronic obstructive pulmonary disease during the day and night increases physical activity additionally.

In further analyses, Westerterp was able to determine that patients lose weight when they exceed a certain level of physical activity. If the energy expenditure for physical activity exceeded 55% of the basal metabolic rate, the patients lost weight.

But if the energy expenditure remained below the 55%, the patients gained weight. This finding is significant as it shows that physical activity in stress is so crucial for weight gain or weight loss.

If an affected person, who is afflicted by the unwanted energy expenditures of the second part of the book during the aging process, still manages to show high physical activity despite the unfavorable circumstances, the body weight will hardly increase but rather fall or at least remain the same. But if the person is forced by the unfavorable circumstances to low physical activity, then there is a risk of weight gain in the concomitant presence of low energy expenditure of the immune system. Finding the balance here is sometimes quite an art.

Weight gain and lower physical activity are then associated with a higher risk of cardiovascular diseases such as heart attack or stroke, metabolic diseases such as diabetes, high blood pressure, depression, and malignant tumors.

References

Block JP, He Y, Zaslavsky AM, Ding L, Ayanian JZ (2009) Psychosocial stress and change in weight among US adults. Am J Epidemiol 170:181–192

Brunner EJ, Chandola T, Marmot MG (2007) Prospective effect of job strain on general and central obesity in the Whitehall II Study. Am J Epidemiol 165:828–837

Da Silva FC, Hernandez SS, Goncalves E, Arancibia BA, Da Silva Castro TL, Da SR (2014) Anthropometric indicators of obesity in policemen: a systematic review of observational studies. Int J Occup Med Environ Health 27:891–901

Dallman MF (2010) Stress-induced obesity and the emotional nervous system. Trends Endocrinol Metab 21:159–165

Hales CN, Barker DJ (2001) The thrifty phenotype hypothesis. Br Med Bull 60:5–20

Hemmingsson E (2014) A new model of the role of psychological and emotional distress in promoting obesity: conceptual review with implications for treatment and prevention. Obes Rev 15:769–779

Hitze B, Hubold C, van DR, Schlichting K, Lehnert H, Entringer S, Peters A (2010) How the selfish brain organizes its supply and demand. Front Neuroenergetics 2:7–17

Hunter GR, Fisher G, Neumeier WH, Carter SJ, Plaisance EP (2015) Exercise Training and Energy Expenditure following Weight Loss. Med Sci Sports Exerc 47:1950–1957

Karelis AD, Lavoie ME, Fontaine J, Messier V, Strychar I, Rabasa-Lhoret R, Doucet E (2010) Anthropometric, metabolic, dietary and psychosocial profiles of underreporters of energy intake: a doubly labeled water study among overweight/obese postmenopausal women--a Montreal Ottawa New Emerging Team study. Eur J Clin Nutr 64:68–74

Kirschbaum C, Prussner JC, Stone AA, Federenko I, Gaab J, Lintz D, Schommer N, Hellhammer DH (1995) Persistent high cortisol responses to repeated psychological stress in a subpopulation of healthy men. Psychosom Med 57:468–474

Korkeila M, Kaprio J, Rissanen A, Koshenvuo M, Sorensen TI (1998) Predictors of major weight gain in adult Finns: stress, life satisfaction and personality traits. Int J Obes Relat Metab Disord 22:949–957

Oliver G, Wardle J (1999) Perceived effects of stress on food choice. Physiol Behav 66:511–515

Organisation für wirtschaftliche Zusammenarbeit und Entwicklung – OECD. Aktuelles Adipositas-Update OECD (im Internet: ▶ http://www.oecd.org/health/obesity-update.htm)

Peters A, McEwen BS (2015) Stress habituation, body shape and cardiovascular mortality. Neurosci Biobehav Rev 56:139–150

Pontzer H, Brown MH, Raichlen DA, Dunsworth H, Hare B, Walker K, Luke A, Dugas LR, Durazo-Arvizu R, Schoeller D, Plange-Rhule J, Bovet P, Forrester TE, Lambert EV, Thompson ME, Shumaker RW, Ross SR (2016) Metabolic acceleration and the evolution of human brain size and life history. Nature 533:390–392

Pontzer H, Raichlen DA, Wood BM, Emery TM, Racette SB, Mabulla AZ, Marlowe FW (2015) Energy expenditure and activity among Hadza hunter-gatherers. Am J Hum Biol 27:628–637

14

References

Redman LM, Kraus WE, Bhapkar M, Das SK, Racette SB, Martin CK, Fontana L, Wong WW, Roberts SB, Ravussin E (2014) Energy requirements in nonobese men and women: results from CALERIE. Am J Clin Nutr 99:71–78

Serlachius A, Hamer M, Wardle J (2007) Stress and weight change in university students in the United Kingdom. Physiol Behav 92:548–553

Stice E, Palmrose CA, Burger KS (2015) Elevated BMI and male sex are associated with greater underreporting of caloric intake as assessed by doubly labeled water. J Nutr 145:2412–2418

St-Onge MP, Roberts AL, Chen J, Kelleman M, O'Keeffe M, RoyChoudhury A, Jones PJ (2011) Short sleep duration increases energy intakes but does not change energy expenditure in normal-weight individuals. Am J Clin Nutr 94:410–416

Westerterp KR (2013) Physical activity and physical activity induced energy expenditure in humans: measurement, determinants, and effects. Front Physiol 4:90

Zizza CA, Duffy PA, Gerrior SA (2008) Food insecurity is not associated with lower energy intakes. Obesity (Silver Spring) 16:1908–1913

The Storage Hormone Insulin Doesn't Work— Insulin Resistance

Contents

15.1   Antonin Sulin in Resistance – 158

15.2   Storage in Chronic Inflammation—Role of Insulin – 158

15.3   Insulin Resistance in Aging – 159

References – 161

© The Author(s), under exclusive license to Springer-Verlag GmbH, DE, part of Springer Nature 2024
R. H. Straub, *Understanding Aging, Fatigue, and Inflammation*,
https://doi.org/10.1007/978-3-662-68904-2_15

15.1 Antonin Sulin in Resistance

Insulin was extensively discussed in ▶ Chap. 1 in relation to energy storage (◘ Fig. 1.8 and ◘ Table 1.3). This hormone of the pancreas is a crucial storage hormone for glucose and fatty acids. Insulin acts on insulin-dependent organs such as muscle and adipose tissue (and liver), promoting the uptake of energy-rich substrates such as glucose and fatty acids. We also learned that pro-inflammatory cytokines like TNF can inhibit the effect of insulin, so cytokines like TNF cause energy release.

The other factors necessary for energy release from the stress axes—noradrenaline, adrenaline, cortisol, growth hormone, thyroid hormones, and the RAA hormones—all inhibit the effect of insulin, this main storage hormone. These factors essentially nullify the effect of insulin directly at the cell by making the cell insensitive or resistant to insulin. We now speak of insulin resistance. Then the uptake of glucose or fatty acids into the storage does not work.

Let us again remember the gas ball from ▶ Chap. 1 "Energy and Body". Imagine a pipe line leading to a western gas ball and transporting gas from Baku on the Caspian Sea. Just before leaving Azerbaijan, there is a gas tap on the pipe line that can shut off the transport. An employee of the Azerbaijan energy company named Antonin Sulin opens the gas tap every morning and closes it every evening. If Antonin has turned off the gas tap in the evening, and he is at a political protest event the next day and therefore in resistance, then no energy will flow and the western gas balls will remain empty. This Antonin-Sulin-Resistance prevents energy flow and energy storage, and this is very similar to insulin and insulin resistance. If Antonin has partied all night (physical stress) or has an infectious disease with high inflammation, he has to stay at home due to illness. He is not in resistance, but the gas tap is still not operated, and the consequences for western gas balls are the same. Nothing is stored.

If we are under stress and the stress axes are activated, or if there is a high inflammation in the body (TNF and other cytokines are high), then **nothing** is stored (Antonin sends his regards). This non-storage happens by switching off the insulin effect.

We also learned that the selfish brain uses the stress axes to demand energy-rich substrates, whereas the selfish immune system uses the pro-inflammatory cytokines to release energy-rich substrates. The two competing realms—brain and immune system—do this in their respective ways by inhibiting the insulin effect (◘ Fig. 3.1, upper half). From these preliminary considerations, one can already guess what will happen in chronic inflammatory diseases with high cytokines.

15.2 Storage in Chronic Inflammation—Role of Insulin

By now, a decrease in insulin action has been observed in various chronic inflammatory diseases that are accompanied by high serum levels of pro-inflammatory cytokines. Insulin is less able to store energy-rich substrates in the storage organs—adipose tissue and muscles. However, this decrease in insulin action only affects the storage organs. The brain and immune system are exempt from this, as these two egoists absorb the energy-rich substrates independently of insulin. They are not storage organs in our body, but energy-consuming organs.

15

This decrease in insulin action is also called insulin resistance, because the storage organs become resistant or insensitive to insulin. In the case of insulin resistance, larger amounts of glucose and fatty acids circulate in the bloodstream, which are brought to the selfish consumers. However, the increased level of glucose in the pancreas leads to an increased secretion of insulin, because the pancreas can and must react directly to the levels of glucose in the blood. High blood glucose is a signal for it to produce even more insulin. This results in a high insulin level, which is called hyperinsulinemia. Thus, it is found that insulin resistance almost always goes hand in hand with hyperinsulinemia. What is the deeper meaning of insulin resistance and hyperinsulinemia?

The matter is basically quite simple. When the effect of insulin on the storage organs decreases, less is stored, and the two egoists get more. Thus, they serve themselves the energy-rich substrates via insulin resistance (◘ Fig. 3.1). Hyperinsulinemia particularly benefits the immune system, as immune cells need insulin as a growth factor. Insulin promotes the growth of immune cells! In the case of immune cells, one should perhaps better say the multiplication of immune cells. This growth or multiplication mechanism was preserved for an acute infectious disease in evolutionary history (positively selected), so that the immune cells that can recognize the pathogen can be multiplied. In the case of an infectious disease, it is therefore advantageous that the stores are emptied and the immune cells can multiply with the help of insulin.

This whole process takes place over a period of 7–14 days during the initial confrontation with an unknown infectious agent. If you're lucky, this machine works perfectly and after 14 days things start to improve. The disease burden decreases, and the immune cells are no longer needed and are discarded. However, if you are dealing with mistakenly recognized, body's own proteins—we called them autoantigens—as in a chronic inflammatory disease, the false game does not end after the usual playing time, but goes into overtime for years and decades. It becomes a chronic inflammatory disease. Now the mechanisms selected for infectious diseases are used again.

The deeper meaning of insulin resistance and hyperinsulinemia then becomes counterproductive, because energy-rich substrates and growth factors are continuously supplied to the mistakenly activated immune system. The immune system is stimulated by this form of hyperinsulinemia. So far, there are no therapies that are based on the inhibition of insulin release or the specific insulin effect on immune cells. The body is too dependent on maintaining normal blood sugar levels, and any therapy in this direction would also unfavorably change blood sugar regulation. However, it would be an interesting therapeutic principle if one could specifically prevent the insulin effect on immune cells.

15.3 Insulin Resistance in Aging

As we age, unwanted energy expenditure and therefore lack of physical activity can lead to weight gain. ◘ Figure 14.2 in the preceding ▶ Chap. 14 made this clear. In patients with weight gain and low physical activity, the fat mass is significantly increased in relation to muscle mass. In adipose tissue, there is an increasing inflammation, with the so-called visceral fat beneath the abdominal muscles in the abdominal cavity being particularly inflammatory. The fat on arms, legs, and buttocks, on the other hand, is hardly inflammatory. The increasing inflammatory activity is then a first trigger for the loss of effectiveness of the storage hormone insulin (leading to insulin resistance).

A second trigger is increasing inactivity, as the ratio of adipose tissue to fat-free tissue becomes unfavorable. In addition, moderate exercise is associated with lower inflammatory activity.

A third trigger is poor nutrition, with high-calorie, energy-dense food rich in sugar and fat promoting the process of hyperinsulinemia. High sugar levels after meals stimulate high insulin levels. High insulin levels and high sugar levels can then lead to insulin resistance over years.

A fourth trigger is the activation of stress axes outside of physical activity due to unwanted energy expenditure. The stress axes of the selfish brain can promote insulin resistance via stress axis hormones—noradrenaline, adrenaline, cortisol, growth hormone, thyroid hormones, and the RAA hormones. If these stress axes are stimulated outside of physical activity, they lead to the provision of energy-rich substrates such as glucose but also to insulin resistance, and because the pancreas sees a lot of glucose, it produces even more insulin. These mechanisms have been preserved for the acute fight-or-flight response throughout evolution (positively selected), but they are extremely unfavorable in chronic stress.

So, in the aging process, we recognize several factors that can independently but especially together in the sense of the "double hit" lead to insulin resistance and hyperinsulinemia. Unlike in chronic inflammatory diseases, where the activated immune system clearly dominates and cytokines are primarily responsible, insulin resistance and hyperinsulinemia in the aging process depend on many factors. Here, the sum of the various events is effective in an integrative way. ◘ Figure 15.1 shows the different factors.

Interestingly, the inhibition of pro-inflammatory TNF in individuals with chronic inflammatory diseases leads to a significant reduction in insulin resistance and hyperinsulinemia. The same treatment does nothing in obese individuals with insulin resistance, as a mild inflammation is present in these individuals, but is not the sole trigger. There, the therapy must also consider all other factors of ◘ Fig. 15.1.

The situation becomes complicated when, over time, the chronic situation leads to an increasing failure of the pancreas. One must imagine that the various factors in ◘ Fig. 15.1 all lead to an increased provision of energy-rich substrates such as glucose and fatty acids. The pancreas is constantly stimulated and can initially stand up to the higher work load. It produces more and more insulin until production increasingly dries up. Then glucose and fatty acids have a damaging effect and destroy the insulin-producing cells, resulting in absolute insulin deficiency.

In susceptible individuals, which depends on personal genetic makeup, the function of the pancreas is more at risk. In these individuals, a so-called age-related diabetes or type 2 diabetes mellitus can develop over years, which then has to be treated with external insulin administration or other measures. With external insulin administration, one wants to remove the energy-rich substrates such as glucose from the bloodstream, but this exacerbates the immune-activating hyperinsulinemia.

15

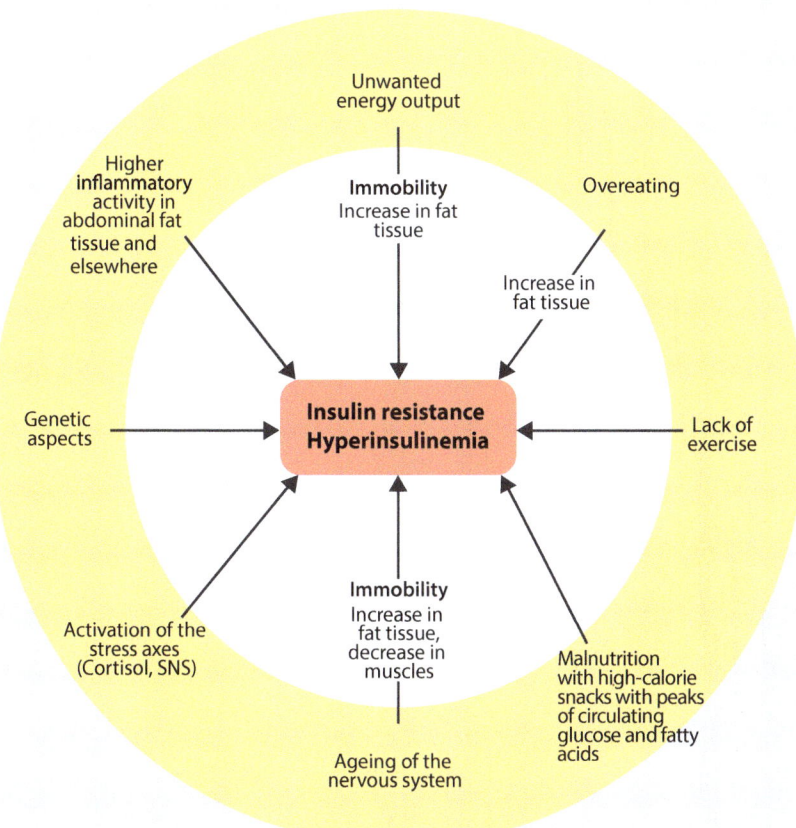

Factors that can lead to insulin resistance and hyperinsulinemia. The unwanted energy expenditures mentioned were discussed in Book Part II. These include inflammation, smoldering inflammation, pain, psychological stress [e.g. care giving or dementia], anxiety, sleep problems, too much smoking, etc.
Abbreviations: SNS, sympathetic nervous system

■ **Fig. 15.1** Factors that can lead to insulin resistance and hyperinsulinemia

Age-related diabetes is the platform for further subsequent problems such as cardio-vascular diseases, heart attack, stroke, etc., which are based on an increased inflammatory situation.

References

Straub RH (2014) Insulin resistance, selfish brain, and selfish immune system: an evolutionarily positively selected program used in chronic inflammatory diseases. Arthritis Res Ther 16(Suppl 2):S4 (pp 1–15)

Decreasing Libido, Lower Fertility

Contents

16.1   Sex and Chronic Inflammation – 164

16.2   Of Antechinus, Sea Elephants, and Macaques – 165

16.3   Estrogens and Chronic Inflammation – 166

16.4   Hormones in Old Age – 167

References – 168

16.1 Sex and Chronic Inflammation

The influence of the selfish immune system on growth, repair, and reproduction has already been discussed in earlier chapters (▶ Chap. 3): "Chronic inflammation also leads to significant disturbances in libido and reproduction. Studies over the last 10 years have shown that even with good anti-inflammatory therapy, disturbances in reproductive functions can still be detected in patients with chronic inflammation. In animal experiments and also in humans, all important reproductive hormones are blocked in the long term during inflammation."

In an impressive experiment conducted at the American National Institute of Health on healthy individuals, the researchers were able to show that the blood levels of the male sex hormone testosterone plummeted massively after a single injection of interleukin-6 (the cytokine or inflammation hormone) (◘ Fig. 16.1). Animal experiments confirmed these findings.

In this experiment, only a small amount of the inflammation factor was injected, and yet the serum levels of the important male sex hormone already dropped to half. In this example, the body only recovered after a week. It is easy to imagine that a more severe and long-term inflammatory situation must lead to a deeper crash and a permanent reduction.

Indeed, in the history of hormone studies in chronic inflammatory diseases, this finding—namely low levels of male sex hormones (androgens)—was the first clearly identifiable hormonal disorder. There was no doubt about it. Already in the 1950s, a Canadian research group was able to observe the low androgen levels. This was later confirmed by various research groups around the world in very different chronic inflammatory diseases, e.g., in the late 1970s by Fehér et al. Finally, the same finding was also observed in **acute** infection or **acute** inflammation.

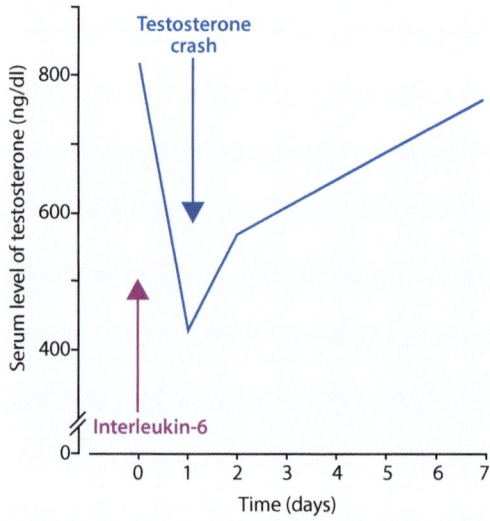

◘ **Fig. 16.1**   Influence of the inflammation factor interleukin-6 on the serum levels of testosterone. (Data from Tsigos et al. 1999)

Low androgen levels are particularly harmful, as androgens play an important role in muscle and bone building and thus in energy and calcium balance, in addition to their reproductive function. The activated and selfish immune system draws on the energy-rich substrates of the muscle (amino acids), no muscle building takes place when an acute infectious disease is present. You will remember that under these circumstances a disease behavior prevails that restricts food intake, so that reserves must be accessed (*Sickness behavior*). The muscle is thus broken down, and reproductive behavior is shut down. In addition, male sex hormones are good inhibitors of the activated immune system. And now the selfishness becomes particularly clear, because it is not the hormonal gland that prevails in acute or chronic inflammation and inhibits the immune system, but the selfish immune system inhibits the endocrine gland because it occupies a hierarchically higher position in the body (see ► Chap. 2 "Evolutionary Medicine").

But why is courtship and reproductive behavior shut down during inflammation?

16.2 Of Antechinus, Sea Elephants, and Macaques

Mating behavior is very energy-consuming, and a striking example can illustrate this. On the Australian continent, there is a pouched mouse named *Antechinus* whose males produce high amounts of testosterone during the peak phase of mating and reproductive behavior, thereby really getting into gear. The males engage in intense mating fights, which is also triggered by higher solar radiation in the Australian summer. During this time, the males move from burrow to burrow, appearing quite agitated but also battered. When it finally comes to copulation, the process can last 12 hours before the exhausted males retreat and die.

The examination of the males shows that they use up all their energy reserves and the immune system no longer functions. The actual cause of death is severe infections with parasites. The selfish brain (reproductive behavior with extremely high psychomotor activity) has dominated in this case, and the immune system has failed. In this way, the male Antechinus live only a single season. They are born in one year, grow rapidly, begin their love life, and then die after continuous copulation (called semelparity). If the males are removed from their habitat in time, they live just as long as the females, 2-3 years.

Another example is provided by northern sea elephants, which are native to the American west coast between California and Alaska. In the males of this species, physical reserves are closely linked to reproductive success. Thick alpha males can go on a long courtship and fight competitive battles because they have many reserves. Because the male sea elephant spends about 160,000 kJ (37,976 kcal) per day during this time. This is 3 times more per day than in the usual life of the sea elephant. The heaviest sea elephants then have the greatest success in terms of offspring. Unlike Antechinus, the male sea elephant has prepared for reproduction through high body weight. If you observe the animals in a documentary, they appear clumsy, but it is extremely effective in terms of reproduction.

The same is true for female macaques observed in Japan. There, reproductive success is also highest when the female monkeys have a high fat weight shortly before the reproductive period. Macaques in Japan have their reproductive period between October and February, so enough fat reserves must be built up during the cold season. If the female monkeys become pregnant on the favorable ground of high fat reserves, they usually have a significantly higher fat weight in the next season, which then again favors reproductive success.

This reminds one of the Barker phenomenon from ▶ Chap. 14 ("Weight changes"), in which fetal energy shortages were held responsible for rapid weight gain. So if female macaques have high fat reserves, get more easily pregnant, and thus create an energy shortage in the fetus (mother as competitor plus cold season), the newborn could better compensate for a lean time if it quickly builds up fat reserves after birth. During their own reproductive phase, such macaque females would then be equipped with higher fat reserves and thus have a higher reproductive success and so on. This is speculation because, to my knowledge, it has not been investigated so far, but it could link the Barker phenomenon with reproductive success.

16.3 Estrogens and Chronic Inflammation

Interestingly, the female sex hormones (estrogens) are less affected by an inflammation-induced crash than the male hormones (androgens)—a phenomenon found in both men and women. This is because male sex hormones (androgens) are converted into estrogens in the area of inflammation. This also occurs in the same way in both men and women. Yes, it is indeed astonishing that the precursors of the female sex hormones are the male sex hormones.

This also applies to hormone production in the ovaries. The estrogens always originate from the androgens and never the other way around, and during inflammation, this conversion is stimulated in the area of inflammation. Thus, the loss of androgens is caused by a lower production in the testes and the adrenal gland and a faster conversion to estrogens in the area of inflammation. Poor men have nothing to laugh about during inflammation, and it is therefore not surprising that chronic inflammatory diseases in men are often more severe than in women.

However, it should be immediately added that women with chronic inflammatory diseases also show disturbances in hormone functions. This is then rather evident in the control hormones of the pituitary gland. Women have relatively normal levels of estrogens during inflammation, but otherwise, the reproductive system is also disturbed. Even in well-treated young women with chronic inflammatory disease today, fertility can be significantly lower. This is particularly the case when the anti-inflammatory therapy is not well adjusted. In women, the number of ovulations is lower, and in men, sperm production and sperm quality are reduced if the inflammatory disease is not well treated.

These findings clearly indicate that reproductive functions are restricted at the expense of the activated and selfish immune system. While these mechanisms were preserved in the context of short-term infectious diseases or other short stimulations of the immune system in evolution (positively selected), the long-term application of this program in chronic inflammatory diseases is unfavorable.

16.4 **Hormones in Old Age**

When we talk about aging, we usually refer to a period that begins in women with menopause and in men with andropause. In ◘ Fig. 8.2, the 50th year of life was identified as a critical point from the perspective of energy expenditure. In both sexes, hormone production decreases increasingly from the age of 50, with the decline in women being more pronounced and faster than in men. Nevertheless, men also show a significant reduction in androgen production, which is referred to as andropause. In women, this point occurs when the last ova are lost from the ovaries. In men, testicular volume and sperm production decrease.

In this phase, the adrenal glands increasingly take over the production of androgens in both women and men, and these androgens are then converted into other androgens or estrogens as needed in various cells of the body. This conversion can take place in the liver, in adipose tissue, but also in immune cells themselves and in the brain. The two egoists obtain the corresponding sex hormones from the precursors.

In summary: Unlike in an inflammatory disease, the decline in sex hormones during aging is not caused by inflammation, but by the increasing demise of the producing tissue—ovaries and testes.

Under Stone Age living conditions, most people did not get old. It is assumed that the average life expectancy was between 25 and 30 years. Occasionally, someone got very old even when favorable circumstances prevailed (e.g., high hierarchical position in the group), but reproduction in old age was a rarity and the old person was certainly not a hero of reproduction. Thus, our ancestors did not experience menopause or andropause at all. Even our closest relatives, the great apes, do not experience this point in the wild. If great apes are kept and cared for in zoos, menopause or andropause can also be observed in them. From this perspective, it also becomes clear why genes were not positively selected for healthy or perfect aging (beyond this point of menopause or andropause).

We have learned that the adrenal gland can at least partially take over the function of the sex hormone-producing glands in old age. There is an androgen of particular interest. It has the somewhat complicated name "De-Hydro-Epi-Andro-Sterone-Sulfate", which is why we prefer to use the simpler abbreviation DHEAS. DHEAS is an androgen that can be converted into other androgens such as testosterone and estrogens.

If we experience an inflammation like an infectious disease or chronic inflammatory disease after menopause or andropause, the blood level of this hormone drops far down. This shows us that the selfish immune system does not tolerate androgens or their precursors in this constellation. It becomes clear that no muscles and bones should be built up during this time of inflammation, as neither testosterone nor estrogens are produced (see ◘ Fig. 1.8).

However, it is fascinating that the blood level of DHEAS also drops when the unwanted energy expenditures mentioned in the second part of the book take a toll for a longer period. In the case of smoldering inflammations, mild long-term inflammations, long-lasting painful conditions, psychological stress such as family care of a dementia patient, and chronic sleep problems, the blood levels of this hormone are often low. Therefore, the concentration of DHEAS can represent a measure of the previous energy strain. The mentioned conditions either consume energy through an activation of the immune system or the brain/nervous system. Both, the selfish immune system and the selfish brain, prevent the production of androgens even during aging, and muscle building or even reproductive behavior are not in the foreground. In a study, we were able to show that the sympathetic nervous system—the henchman of the selfish brain—is decisively involved in this inhibition of DHEAS.

This also makes it understandable why additional energy expenditure by the immune system or brain during aging pose a problem for the muscles. Some doctors therefore suggest taking DHEAS during aging. The author is skeptical at this point for two reasons:

- There are no reliable long-term studies showing that DHEAS can be taken without complications. Short-term studies show few complications. However, since DHEAS can be converted into androgens and estrogens, the usual risks for hormone-dependent diseases such as prostate cancer and breast/uterus cancer exist with long-term use.
- DHEAS is not the only hormone that declines in old age and under the mentioned energy strain. So we would probably have to replace many hormones, and there are no reasonable studies for this. Since the situation is much more complex, the replacement of a single hormone is questionable.

References

Baur M, Ziegler G (2001) Die Odyssee des Menschen – Es begann in Afrika. Econ Ullstein List Verlag, München

Crocker DE, Houser DS, Webb PM (2012) Impact of body reserves on energy expenditure, water flux, and mating success in breeding male northern elephant seals. Physiol Biochem Zool 85:11–20

Feher GK, Feher T, Zahumenszky Z (1979) Study on the inactivation mechanism of androgens in rheumatoid arthritis: excretory rate of free and conjugated 17-ketosteroids. Endokrinologie 73:167–172

Howard RP, Venning EH, Fisk GH (1950). Rheumatoid arthritis. II. Studies of adrenocortical and hypophyseal function and the effects thereon of testosterone and pregnenolone therapy. Can Med Assoc J. 63:340–342

Kizildere S, Glück T, Zietz B, Schölmerich J, Straub RH (2003). During a corticotropin-releasing hormone test in healthy subjects, administration of a beta-adrenergic antagonist induced secretion of cortisol and dehydroepiandrosterone sulfate and inhibited secretion of ACTH. Eur J Endocrinol. 148:45–53

Straub RH (2015) The origin of chronic inflammatory systemic diseases and their sequelae. Academic Press, San Diego

Tsigos C, Papanicolaou DA, Kyrou I, Raptis SA, Chrousos GP (1999) Dose-dependent effects of recombinant human interleukin-6 on the pituitary-testicular axis. J Interferon Cytokine Res 19:1271–1276

Sympathetic Nervous System Fires and Causes High Blood Pressure

Contents

17.1   Cortisol and Inflammation – 170

17.2   Cooperation of Stress Hormones and Consequence in Chronic Inflammation – 171

17.3   Sympathetic Nervous System and Aging – 173

17.4   Low Activity of the Parasympathetic Nervous System – 173

       References – 175

© The Author(s), under exclusive license to Springer-Verlag GmbH, DE, part of Springer Nature 2024
R. H. Straub, *Understanding Aging, Fatigue, and Inflammation*,
https://doi.org/10.1007/978-3-662-68904-2_17

In Book Part I and there in ▣ Fig. 3.1 the role of the sympathetic nervous system and its neurotransmitters adrenaline and noradrenaline for the release of stored energy was shown. If the selfish brain takes a dominant role, it activates the sympathetic nervous system, and the cortisol-producing hormone axis of the pituitary gland and adrenal glands, to release glucose and fatty acids above all and to benefit from them. On the other hand, if the selfish immune system is activated in the short term, it also stimulates the sympathetic nervous system and the cortisol stress axis, which in ▶ Chap. 3 "Brain and Immune System—Two Competing Empires" was called mutual immediate assistance, because the brain helps out in the short term.

It should be noted here that the activity of the sympathetic nervous system also decisively determines blood pressure (high activity means high blood pressure). In the long-term inflammation process, however, the behavior of the two stress axes changes increasingly. There is a normalization or exhaustion of the cortisol stress axis and a noticeable increase in the activity of the sympathetic nervous system.

17.1 Cortisol and Inflammation

Since inflammation is an energy-consuming process, it should not last too long. Usual acute inflammatory diseases such as infections affect us for 1–14 days, maybe 3 weeks. While within 1–3 days the increased inflammatory situation of the selfish immune system calls on the brain for "mutual immediate assistance", the systems change with increasing duration of the disease. The brain goes into the mode of *Sickness behavior*—it basically exits—and the immune system dominates the selfish game outside the brain in the body periphery (at the sites of inflammation).

We observe a normalization of the initially increased activity of the cortisol stress axis after a few days, so that even with high inflammation, quasi normal to reduced values for cortisol in the serum can be measured. The same exhaustion was shown in the 1990s in patients with tumor disease after multiple injections of interleukin-6—the well-known messenger of the immune system. The patients initially showed a strong reaction of the cortisol stress axis with high blood levels of cortisol on day 1 and also 1–2 days afterwards. However, the reaction increasingly exhausted when interleukin-6 was injected over 3 weeks.

Very similar findings were obtained by a Viennese working group with another immune messenger. Initially, there was a strong immediate reaction of the cortisol stress axis, which significantly exhausted after 3 weeks, although the same amount of the messenger substance was injected. Today we know that various messengers of the immune system inhibit the stress axis of the pituitary gland and the adrenal glands with chronic use. Something similar also happens with chronic inflammatory disease.

But what is the deeper meaning of this inhibition?

Cortisol is on the one hand a hormone that can release energy-rich substrates such as glucose from the liver, fatty acids from the adipose tissue and amino acids from the muscle. On the other hand, as a hormone of a brain stress axis, it is capable of massively inhibiting the immune system. Cortisol—similar to the glucocorticoids used in therapy (the layman says cortisone)—is the strongest endogenous inhibitor of the immune system. Cortisol is the hormone that paralyzes the immune system. It is the weapon of the selfish brain to outplay the selfish immune system. So if there would be a long-term increase of this hormone in an infectious disease, i.e. a continuous increase over many days and weeks beyond the "mutual immediate assistance" of the brain, one would not survive an infectious disease. The immune system would be blocked, the pathogens would multiply, and one would die of sepsis.

The immune system must not be continuously inhibited in this situation, because the corresponding countermeasures of the immune cells against the pathogen would not work. In this respect, a program for normalization or exhaustion of the cortisol stress axis despite continuously increased activity of the immune system is valuable. Exactly this happens within a week with continuous use of immune messengers like interleukin-6, as described above.

In patients with chronic inflammatory diseases, something similar happens. The cortisol stress axis exhausts and cortisol does not work well in immune cells due to cortisol resistance.

17.2 Cooperation of Stress Hormones and Consequence in Chronic Inflammation

Since cortisol has several important functions throughout the body, its failure is unfavorable. For example, cortisol, along with noradrenaline and adrenaline, is involved in the stabilization of blood pressure. This can be observed, for example, when patients with sepsis develop circulatory shock. In the case of circulatory shock, noradrenaline/adrenaline is usually used to stabilize blood pressure. However, if these two neurotransmitters no longer help sufficiently, cortisol is additionally given, which then enhances the effect of noradrenaline/adrenaline. This shows the cooperation.

In addition, cortisol and noradrenaline/adrenaline also work together to supply the body with glucose from the liver. We already learned this in Book Part I, ▶ Chap. 1 ("Stress hormones and cytokines release energy"). Furthermore, the three hormones work together to regulate the width of the bronchi in the lungs, where they are responsible for opening the bronchi. Asthmatics therefore often take preparations that open the bronchi like adrenaline, and at the same time they take a cortisol preparation for exactly the same purpose. The substances reinforce each other, and together they open the bronchi much more effectively.

This cooperation of the stress hormones cortisol and noradrenaline/adrenaline is therefore very important, and that's why they also follow the same circadian rhythm, as shown in ▶ Chap. 10, ▣ Fig. 10.3. The hormones help each other, and it now also becomes clear why a one-sided inhibition of the cortisol stress axis may cause a shift to a higher activity of the sympathetic nervous system. Thus, the sympathetic nervous system does not become sluggish in the same way as the cortisol stress axis during long-term inflammation. On the contrary, it has to compensate for this lack of cooperation from cortisol. If one slackens, the other participant has to do more.

The sympathetic nervous system therefore becomes more active, and this can be observed in patients with chronic inflammatory diseases. Some studies on patients with rheumatoid arthritis, the juvenile form of arthritis, and other chronic inflammatory diseases show a higher activity of the sympathetic nervous system with normal to a somewhat reduced cortisol stress axis.

Since the RAA hormones for stabilizing blood pressure—we got to know them in Book Part I in ► Chap. 1 under "Stress hormones and cytokines release energy"—are also stimulated by the sympathetic nervous system, several factors come into play under these new conditions of chronic inflammation that increase blood pressure. The neurotransmitters noradrenaline/adrenaline and the RAA hormones do this by constricting the vessels, by increasing the water within the vessels, and by inhibiting water excretion in the kidneys.

A constriction plus more water volume in the vascular system creates higher pressure. The blood pressure increases. Is this just a accident of inflammation, or does it have a deeper meaning?

We learned from evolutionary medicine that the physiological processes with an activation of the immune system were essentially conserved for a short-term inflammatory reaction in case of injury or infection (were positively selected). So we need to look exactly there, at the infection, if we want to recognize a deeper meaning of a blood pressure increase in inflammation.

Infectious diseases often go hand in hand with water loss due to sweating in fever, increased breathing (water is lost with the exhaled air), diarrhea, vomiting, loss of wound fluid and other fluids. So if the normal water loss via the kidney is inhibited during an infectious disease, this is advantageous because it is lost elsewhere. During an infectious disease, the intake of food, but also of fluids, is also restricted due to *Sickness behavior*.

Remember your highly concentrated urine during the last episode of an infectious disease. This is the sign of a low water excretion, and this blockade is valuable. The sympathetic nervous system and the RAA hormones do exactly this. They inhibit water excretion in the kidney. But what happens when these hormones are activated and no water loss is observed?

In chronic inflammatory disease, a similar mechanism is switched on by the immune messenger substances (interleukin-6 and others), but the water loss is not or hardly increased. So there must be a problem with vasoconstriction and inhibition of water excretion. And indeed: In patients with inflammatory diseases, a higher water volume in the body and a higher blood pressure are found. Since both factors, in addition to inflammatory factors, are held responsible for a higher number of cardiovascular diseases (stroke, heart attack), this mechanism, which was preserved for short-term infectious diseases in our evolutionary history (was positively selected), is unfavorable in chronic inflammatory diseases.

In chronic inflammatory diseases, mortality is still slightly increased compared to the general population, even though the inhibition of inflammation through medication has become very effective. The slightly increased premature mortality is primarily caused by cardiovascular diseases such as stroke and heart attack. If we now consider the mechanisms described above, we also understand why hypertension, cardiovascular diseases, and mortality are still somewhat more prevalent. In the future, in addition to controlling inflammation, hypertension and cardiovascular diseases must necessarily become much more the focus of interest.

17

17.3 Sympathetic Nervous System and Aging

Even during aging, the activity of the sympathetic nervous system constantly increases. In contrast, the cortisol stress axis remains about the same. Both stress hormones increase significantly in relation to the sex hormones, with the neurotransmitters of the sympathetic nervous system dominating above all.

This situation strongly reminds us of chronic inflammatory diseases, and one wonders whether the same mechanisms play a role. We have learned that inflammation increases during aging. This is particularly the case under stressful life events, as ◘ Fig. 4.2 illustrates under "Strength of Inflammation". We also repeatedly asked ourselves whether the slightly increased inflammation in old age *alone* is sufficient to stimulate the various problems mentioned in Book Part III. This was generally denied for the situation during aging, and the other factors with undesirably increased energy expenditure were held responsible. They were considered because they reduced the desired energy expenditures for physical activity.

In fact, these mentioned undesirable factors all contribute to an increase in the activity of the stress axes, but especially of the sympathetic nervous system. This should not surprise us at all, because we have learned that a higher energy expenditure can only be guaranteed if energy-rich substrates such as glucose and fatty acids can be provided. Who provides them? These are the stress axes with noradrenaline/adrenaline and cortisol or the immune system with its cytokines. Undesirable factors are associated with higher energy expenditure, and this demands a higher activity of the energy-providing stress axes.

Other phenomena that lead to an increase in the sympathetic nervous system are physical activities. However, if we are confronted with sympathetic nervous system-stimulating activities due to a generally poorer training situation with reduced physical activity because of the undesirable other energy expenditures, the response of the sympathetic nervous system is often excessive—adrenaline and noradrenaline increase in the blood more than necessary. In trained people, the sympathetic nervous system responds appropriately, the activity goes up a bit, and normal state is quickly restored. This is different in untrained people, because the activity increases strongly and remains high for a long time. There is an overcompensation there.

For these reasons, not only a slightly increasing inflammation during aging, but also the other undesirable energy expenditures influence the activity of the sympathetic nervous system. High blood pressure during aging can also be contributed to by direct changes in the kidneys and their hormone system and the arterial vessel walls (kidney-specific diseases and vascular diseases). These last points are not further discussed under the chapter heading.

17.4 Low Activity of the Parasympathetic Nervous System

When talking about the sympathetic nervous system, one must always also talk about the parasympathetic nervous system, as they mutually influence each other. They are important adversaries. This consideration could have been discussed in a separate chapter, but due to the direct relationship with the sympathetic nervous system, it is briefly mentioned here. If the activity of the sympathetic nervous system is increased, the activity of the parasympathetic nervous system is reduced.

Essential tasks of the parasympathetic nervous system concern the vagus nerve, which we have extensively learned about in energy storage in ▶ Chap. 1, for example in ◘ Figs. 1.7, 1.8 and ◘ Table 1.3. This important nerve primarily has digestive functions, so it is crucially involved in food intake. In addition, the vagus nerve stimulates insulin secretion and thus contributes to the storage of energy-rich substrates. Then, the vagus nerve is responsible for lowering the heart rate and thus takes on exactly opposite functions to the sympathetic nervous system.

In the context of an acute inflammatory disease, the function of the parasympathetic nervous system is blocked, food intake is reduced, digestive function is throttled, the stimulating influences on insulin release are reduced, in short, in this constellation the sympathetic nervous system is activated, and the energy-rich substrates are released from the stores. We discussed that a similar constellation is found in chronic inflammatory diseases, which ultimately contributes to inflammation-related loss of appetite. In chronic inflammatory diseases, it has been clearly shown that parasympathetic function is reduced. This is no surprise if the sympathetic nerve function is increased.

In recent years, the importance of the vagus nerve for acute inflammation has been examined more closely. It could be shown that the vagus has an anti-inflammatory effect. Most publications on this topic have mainly examined acute inflammatory conditions. And there it is indeed the case: "The vagus causes an inflammation inhibition."

However, it remains unclear whether this parasympathetic function can also play a role in chronic inflammatory diseases. Since the parasympathetic nervous system is less active in chronic inflammatory diseases, the associated inflammation inhibition is probably less effective. Advocates of this theory imagine that chronic inflammation can be inhibited by electrical stimulation of the vagus nerve, although this electrical stimulation has so far only been partially successful in a few patients with chronic inflammatory diseases with non-blinded study conditions.

Also during the aging process, in which the activity of the sympathetic nervous system increases, the function of the vagus nerve increasingly decreases. There are several indications for this declining function, which can be particularly well observed in the heart rate and heart rate variability. High variability is coupled with a parasympathetic function, and this decreases with aging. Sleep disorders reduce parasympathetic and increase sympathetic activity. High body weight is associated with lower parasympathetic activity and higher sympathetic nerve activity. Many stressful activities are associated with lower parasympathetic activity. The reduced parasympathetic activity also becomes visible in the form of increasing digestive problems in old age, as the vagus nerve is significantly involved in this.

The parasympathetic function can be positively influenced by endurance training and weight loss, and these measures also reduce sympathetic activity. Once again: Being physically active is beneficial.

17

References

Bruchfeld A, Goldstein RS, Chavan S, Patel NB, Rosas-Ballina M, Kohn N, Qureshi AR, Tracey KJ (2010) Whole blood cytokine attenuation by cholinergic agonists ex vivo and relationship to vagus nerve activity in rheumatoid arthritis. J Intern Med 268:94–101

Gisslinger H, Svoboda T, Clodi M, Gilly B, Ludwig H, Havelec L, Luger A (1993) Interferon-alpha stimulates the hypothalamic-pituitary-adrenal axis in vivo and in vitro. Neuroendocrinology 57:489–495

Günther F, Ehrenstein B, Hartung W, Boschiero D, Fleck M, Straub RH (2021). Increased extracellular water measured by bioimpedance analysis and increased serum levels of atrial natriuretic peptide in polymyalgia rheumatica patients: Signs of volume overload. Z Rheumatol. 80:140–148

Mastorakos G, Chrousos GP, Weber JS (1993) Recombinant interleukin-6 activates the hypothalamic-pituitary-adrenal axis in humans. J Clin Endocrinol Metab 77:1690–1694

Sloan RP, McCreath H, Tracey KJ, Sidney S, Liu K, Seeman T (2007) RR interval variability is inversely related to inflammatory markers: the CARDIA study. Mol Med 13:178–184

Spath-Schwalbe E, Porzsolt F, Digel W, Born J, Kloss B, Fehm HL (1989) Elevated plasma cortisol levels during interferon-gamma treatment. Immunopharmacology 17:141–145

Straub RH (2012) Evolutionary medicine and chronic inflammatory state – known and new concepts in pathophysiology. J Mol Med 90:523–534

Straub RH, Cutolo M, Zietz B, Schölmerich J (2001) The process of aging changes the interplay of the immune, endocrine and nervous systems. Mech Ageing Dev 122:1591–1611

Straub RH, Ehrenstein B, Gunther F, Rauch L, Trendafilova N, Boschiero D, Grifka J, Fleck M (2017) Increased extracellular water measured by bioimpedance and by increased serum levels of atrial natriuretic peptide in RA patients-signs of volume overload. Clin Rheumatol 36:1041–1051

Thayer JF, Yamamoto SS, Brosschot JF (2010) The relationship of autonomic imbalance, heart rate variability and cardiovascular disease risk factors. Int J Cardiol 141:122–131

Increased Blood Clotting—Thrombosis/Embolism

Contents

18.1   Coagulation Explained: Lampreys, Sea Squirts, Fugu, and Humans – 178

18.2   Coagulation and Inflammation – 180

18.3   Increased Coagulation in Chronic Inflammation – 181

18.4   Acceleration of Coagulation in Old Age – 182

References – 182

© The Author(s), under exclusive license to Springer-Verlag GmbH, DE, part of Springer Nature 2024
R. H. Straub, *Understanding Aging, Fatigue, and Inflammation*,
https://doi.org/10.1007/978-3-662-68904-2_18

18.1 Coagulation Explained: Lampreys, Sea Squirts, Fugu, and Humans

The topic is discussed here because blood coagulation is an important factor in the context of evolutionary medicine, but also in heart attack, stroke, pulmonary embolism, and inflammation. There is also a direct relationship between blood coagulation and energy balance.

Blood coagulation became vital when the first tubular vascular systems for the transport of oxygen and energy carriers appeared on the stage of evolution. In a very appealing book, Russell Doolittle, a biochemist at the University of San Diego, describes the evolution of blood coagulation over 500 million years (it is a biochemical textbook, although he wanted to write a book for the general public).

It is made clear that our very distant ancestors, such as the jawless lampreys (*Petromyzontiformes*), but also the sessile sea squirts (*Ascidiacea*) already have important blood coagulation factors in their vascular system, which have a great similarity with the corresponding blood coagulation factors of humans. When the jaw-bearing bony fish like the puffer fish (*Tetraodontidae*)—for example the Japanese food fish named Fugu—entered the stage 450 million years ago, almost all the coagulation factors known to us today had developed in these animals. We seal our vessels with the same factors as the poisonous puffer fish.

The sealing of vessels in case of vascular injuries is a primary task, as life with blood-transporting tubular systems without this blood coagulation function is unthinkable. ◘ Figure 18.1 schematically shows the mechanisms of blood coagulation. Injury and bleeding are acute events, which require an immediate response from blood coagulation. Now one can ask under what circumstances injuries occur, and one will soon come across fight and/or flight situations.

Under natural living conditions—the Pygmies in Cameroon or the Hadza in Tanzania—vascular injury in combat is an important factor. The most common cause of death in today's warfare is gunshot or explosion injuries with large bleedings. If fight and/or flight reactions are directly associated with vascular injuries or blood coagulation, it is now hardly surprising that the sympathetic nervous system plays a very important role in blood coagulation.

The sympathetic nervous system can promote but also inhibit blood coagulation via the two hormones adrenaline and noradrenaline. It is important to know that blood coagulation forms a very complex system of coagulation-promoting and coagulation-inhibiting factors. The balance between the two sides is crucial, and this balance must be shifted towards blood coagulation at a site with vascular injury (◘ Fig. 18.1). Otherwise, the system must be kept in balance, otherwise there would be coagulation within the vessels (◘ Fig. 18.1). There are indeed disease states where this happens in the vessel, but this situation is often fatal.

Thus, adrenaline can particularly lead to an activation of the coagulation-promoting side when components of the vessel walls or the surrounding tissue are exposed that would not be present without injury (◘ Fig. 18.1). Under these circumstances, adrenaline activates the platelets so that they can aggregate better. So if the inner wall of the vessel is damaged, then the hormones of the sympathetic nervous system are strong promoters of blood coagulation at the site of damage.

18

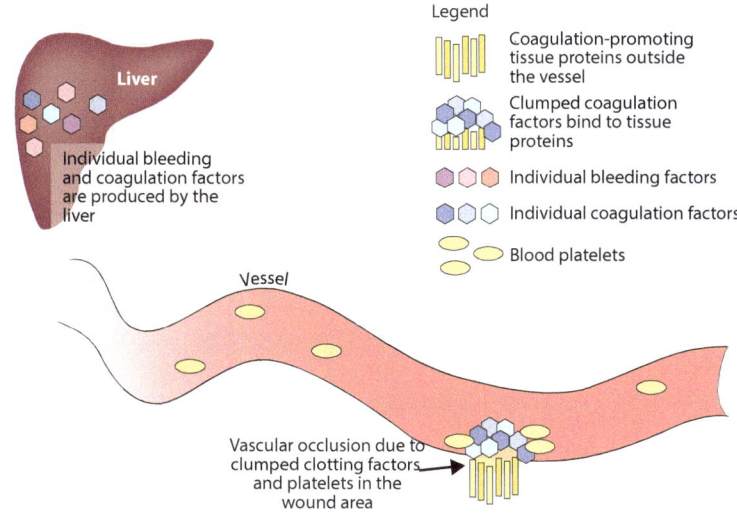

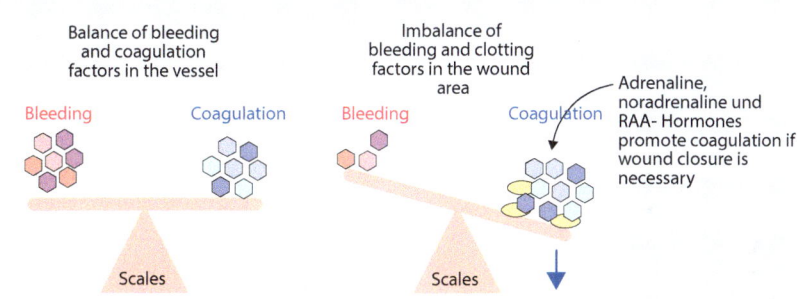

Blood coagulation in the human body. There are coagulation and bleeding factors that are produced in the liver (a) and that must be in balance in the vascular system in the flowing blood (b, left). The bleeding factors are antagonists of the coagulation factors, which are particularly important in the healthy and uninjured vascular system (b, left) in order to prevent coagulation. Small micro-injuries to the vascular wall occur again and again, and this is precisely where the bleeding factors are important, so that excessive coagulation in the vascular system does not occur every time. When a vascular wound occurs, coagulation factors and blood platelets come into direct contact with tissue proteins that promote coagulation (a). This contact triggers a chain reaction that leads to a clot and seals the vessel (a and b, right). The coagulation factors outweigh the bleeding factors (b).

Abbreviation:
RAA = blood pressure hormones such as renin, angiotensin, aldosterone

■ **Fig. 18.1**   Blood coagulation in the human body

In a real "fight situation", for example during and after a marathon run and up to 21 hours afterwards, both coagulation-promoting and coagulation-inhibiting factors are increasingly formed. Furthermore, under such circumstances, platelets are activated, which are needed for immediate sealing. If there is no damage to the inner wall of the vessel in such a marathon runner, there is no blood coagulation.

In ◘ Fig. 18.1 it was shown that coagulation only occurs when the coagulation factors present in the vessel come into direct contact with coagulation-promoting tissue proteins. This happens, for example, in the case of a wound. So if there is a vascular damage or injury, then the sympathetic nervous system with adrenaline promotes blood coagulation on site.

Another important hormone system that promotes blood coagulation are the blood pressure-stabilizing RAA hormones, which we have come to know in the context of energy release and blood pressure increase (▶ Chap. 17 "Sympathetic fires and causes high blood pressure"). These RAA hormones are activated by the sympathetic nervous system. Since a vascular injury with blood loss requires not only blood coagulation but also blood pressure stabilization and tissue repair, it is no longer surprising that these connections between sympathetic nervous system, RAA hormones, blood coagulation, and energy provision exist.

Under favorable circumstances, blood clotting only occurs where it is necessary—namely in the vascular wound area (◘ Fig. 18.1). However, if there are already minor damages to the inner wall of the vessel and the normally hidden components of the vessel walls or surrounding tissue are exposed, there is a risk of local formation of a blood clot and the detachment of the blood clot from the vessel wall, which can appear as an embolism.

18.2 Coagulation and Inflammation

Another situation with changes in vascular permeability is inflammation, because in inflammation the walls of very small vessels generally become more permeable. This increased permeability has the advantage that immune cells flowing in the vessel can pass through the wall more easily. If an infection-related inflammatory process takes place near a vessel, the facilitated passage of immune cells is valuable. However, this can also increase the risk of bleeding. It is therefore not surprising that inflammatory factors such as the cytokines already mentioned (Interleukin-6 or TNF) can increase the coagulation activity of the blood.

The blood clotting factors are directly involved in the elimination of infectious pathogens in the wound area. Blood clotting factors activate immune cells and vice versa, so that microbes can be eliminated more quickly. The clot also serves to isolate the pathogens within the clot. Clotting factors stimulate other cells to produce endogenous antibiotics. Mice that cannot produce a clotting factor are more susceptible to infections with bacteria. Mice that clot more because they lack a bleeding factor are better protected against bacterial infections. Blood clotting factors are involved in the formation of new vessels in an inflammatory area or wound area, so that more immune cells can be attracted. So there is a clear connection between blood clotting and infection defense.

The important connection to energy balance is shown in the infobox "Explanation".

Explanation: Blood clotting and Energy expenditure

Bleeding can be associated with a large loss of cellular components of the blood, especially red blood cells. The production of red blood cells and other lost factors is an expensive business. This can be seen particularly when looking at hereditary diseases of the blood formation system. Children with a so-called sickle cell anemia, in which the red blood cells are not correctly produced, have a high turnover of red blood cells. The body constantly destroys the pathological red blood cells and continuously produces new, but pathological ones, to compensate for the deficiency situation. This situation also arises after blood loss due to injury or wounding.

A person with sickle cell anemia has a daily energy expenditure that is about 16% higher—by the way, a completely unwanted energy expenditure. This corresponds with a daily energy expenditure of 10,000 kJ (2,388 kcal) to about 1,600 kJ (382 kcal) more per day. If you convert this into physical activity, you could dance for an hour or cycle for 35 minutes.

It is therefore not surprising that the energy release system from the sympathetic nervous system, the cortisol stress axis and others is activated during bleeding.

18.3 Increased Coagulation in Chronic Inflammation

When we now consider chronic inflammatory diseases, in which the sympathetic nervous system and the RAA hormones are more active, and in which inflammation factors such as interleukin-6 or TNF are increased, it does not surprise us at all if coagulation is also more strongly activated in these patients. Once again: The mechanisms that come into play in chronic inflammatory diseases were conserved during evolutionary history in the context of acute infections (positively selected).

As early as the 1940s, it was found that patients with rheumatoid arthritis showed altered blood coagulation. This finding has been confirmed multiple times in this disease, but also in other chronic inflammatory diseases. In this context, the coagulation system, but also the anti-coagulation system, is more active. The balance between coagulation-promoting and coagulation-inhibiting factors is thus maintained, but everything is active at a higher level.

When additional factors such as vascular wall damage occur, exposing structures that are normally not present, there is a risk of local formation of a blood clot. Within the inflammation area in the joint, these additional factors are often openly exposed. There is also a higher coagulability, as one would expect if infectious agents had penetrated there and needed to be eliminated and sealed off in a plug.

In a published study in patients with rheumatoid arthritis, the authors were able to show that interleukin-6 is associated with a blood coagulation-promoting situation. The authors treated the patients with an inhibitor of interleukin-6 and were then able to observe that the coagulation-promoting factors decreased. Very similar findings were observed in these patients after inhibition of TNF. These studies very impressively demonstrate the altered coagulation situation in these patients.

So if we assume increased blood coagulation, it is not surprising that the risk of a heart attack, stroke, or embolism is increased. These factors also contribute to increased premature mortality, in addition to the points mentioned above. If we are aware of these points, we will need to conduct therapy studies in the future to improve this situation in patients with chronic inflammatory diseases.

18.4 Acceleration of Coagulation in Old Age

During the aging process, the risk of heart attacks, strokes, embolisms, and thromboses—diseases with increased blood coagulation—increases, and therefore similar processes as in chronic inflammatory diseases could play a role. It has already been reported that the activity of the sympathetic nervous system increases and that the inflammation situation slightly increases during aging. We are also increasingly affected by stressful life circumstances (Book Part II "Energy Expenditures in the Spotlight"), which in turn activate the sympathetic nervous system and promote inflammation. Both factors could mean an increase in blood coagulation. In detail, it has indeed been shown that several coagulation-promoting factors increase during aging. The sympathetic nervous system plays a promoting role in this.

Some studies also suggest that fat cells of the abdominal fat tissue can produce important coagulation-promoting factors. Thus, an increase in abdominal fat tissue, which has already been discussed in this book, would be another important factor that stimulates blood coagulation in old age.

Furthermore, the nature of the vessel walls changes during aging, leading to an altered function of the inner vessel wall and to an increasing vessel thickness and stiffness. Both factors can promote the coagulation process, especially in the area of a pre-damaged wall. In addition, during aging, there is an increasing narrowing of the vessels, leading to higher blood pressure and higher shear forces. The sympathetic nervous system plays an important role in this again.

It has been shown that physical activity (aerobic endurance training and resistance training) reduces these problems. With moderate training, coagulation-promoting factors are lowered and vascular-related problems are reduced. It would therefore prove useful again if unwanted energy expenditures could be reduced and desired energy reserves could be made available for physical activity.

References

Dimitroulas T, Douglas KM, Panoulas VF, Toms T, Smith JP, Treharne GJ, Nightingale P, Hodson J, Kitas GD (2013) Derangement of hemostasis in rheumatoid arthritis: association with demographic, inflammatory and metabolic factors. Clin Rheumatol 32:1357–1364

Doolittle RF (2012) Stanching the flow: The evolution of vertebrate blood clotting. University Science Books, Mill Valley, California

Fiusa MM, Carvalho-Filho MA, Annichino-Bizzacchi JM, De Paula EV (2015) Causes and consequences of coagulation activation in sepsis: an evolutionary medicine perspective. BMC Med 13:105–327

Gualtierotti R, Ingegnoli F, Griffini S, Grovetti E, Meroni PL, Cugno M (2016) Prothrombotic biomarkers in patients with rheumatoid arthritis: the beneficial effect of IL-6 receptor blockade. Clin Exp Rheumatol 34:451–458

18

Ingegnoli F, Fantini F, Griffini S, Soldi A, Meroni PL, Cugno M (2010) Anti-tumor necrosis factor alpha therapy normalizes fibrinolysis impairment in patients with active rheumatoid arthritis. Clin Exp Rheumatol 28:254–257

Lucchesi O, Lucchesi M, Bailonie S (1946) Weltmann coagulation reaction in rheumatoid arthritis. Ann Rheum Dis 5:78–82

Otowa K, Takamura M, Murai H, Maruyama M, Nakano M, Ikeda T, Kobayashi D, Ootsuji H, Okajima M, Furushou H, Yuasa T, Takata S, Kaneko S (2008) Altered interaction between plasminogen activator inhibitor type 1 activity and sympathetic nerve activity with aging. Circ J 72:458–462

Seals DR, Desouza CA, Donato AJ, Tanaka H (2008) Habitual exercise and arterial aging. J Appl Physiol (1985) 105:1323–1332

Straub RH (2015) The origin of chronic inflammatory systemic diseases and their sequelae. Academic, San Diego

van den Oever IA, Sattar N, Nurmohamed MT (2014) Thromboembolic and cardiovascular risk in rheumatoid arthritis: role of the haemostatic system. Ann Rheum Dis 73:954–957

van der Poll T, Herwald H (2014) The coagulation system and its function in early immune defense. Thromb Haemost 112:640–648

von Kanel R, Kudielka BM, Abd-el-Razik A, Gander ML, Frey K, Fischer JE (2004) Relationship between overnight neuroendocrine activity and morning haemostasis in working men. Clin Sci (Lond) 107:89–95

Yamamoto K, Takeshita K, Saito H (2014) Plasminogen activator inhibitor-1 in aging. Semin Thromb Hemost 40:652–659

Stress Worsens Inflammation, and Inflammation Alters Stress Tolerance

Contents

19.1   Stress and Factor X Constitute a Double Hit – 2

19.2   Anti-Stress Therapies – 3

19.3   Stress in the Elderly – 4

References – 6

© The Author(s), under exclusive license to Springer-Verlag GmbH, DE, part of Springer Nature 2024
R. H. Straub, *Understanding Aging, Fatigue, and Inflammation*,
https://doi.org/10.1007/978-3-662-68904-2_19

There is acute and chronic stress. Chronic stress is experienced when caring for family members (*Caregiver-Stress*), dementia diseases such as Parkinson's, childhood adverse experiences (example: severe illness and death of a parent), severe stressful life events in adulthood (example: war experiences or natural disasters), chronic diseases such as heart failure, loneliness especially in old age, disputes at the workplace and much more. Chronic stress is associated with an increased energy expenditure on the order of 10–35% above the control level of unstressed individuals.

It has already been reported that stress is also linked to an activation of the immune system, and as an example, the *Caregiver-Stress* when caring for a family member was mentioned (■ Fig. 4.2). The interleukin-6 in the serum was increased in the *Caregiver*. Another important point was the ominous convergence of stress and an inflammatory disease, which can exacerbate the problems. The following text will now discuss this relationship in detail in the case of chronic inflammatory diseases.

19.1 Stress and Factor X Constitute a Double Hit

In patients with chronic inflammatory diseases such as rheumatoid arthritis, stress has an inflammation-promoting component. We can even go so far as to say that stress promotes the disease flare-ups that repeatedly occur in these diseases. In individual cases—for example in the juvenile form of arthritis—a direct connection between stress in childhood and later onset of the disease was found in studies. Stress leads to measurably higher blood levels of cytokines such as interleukin-1, interleukin-6, TNF and others in these diseases. But one wonders how this practically happens.

In the last 10–15 years, it has been possible to find important genetic factors that play a crucial role in the occurrence of chronic inflammatory diseases. This includes Factor X, which is necessary for switching off an inflammatory cell reaction. For example, when an immune cell is stimulated by bacteria, Factor X (see glossary in the appendix) is also stimulated to slow down the inflammatory reaction. Because in addition to the pro-inflammatory factors, there must always be anti-inflammatory factors to maintain balance, and Factor X is such an anti-inflammatory protein in the cell.

If Factor X completely fails in humans, there is a chronic inflammatory disease with arthritis, eye inflammation, small ulcers in the oral cavity and in the genital area etc. This shows us that Factor X generally suppresses inflammation and is therefore very important.

In some chronic inflammatory diseases, a genetic change in Factor X is associated with a reduced function. Since Factor X acts anti-inflammatory, a reduced function means "stronger inflammation". Thus, in some patients with rheumatoid arthritis but also in psoriasis, multiple sclerosis, diabetes mellitus in young adulthood (called type 1 diabetes mellitus) and other chronic inflammatory diseases, a disturbed Factor X can be a genetic characteristic. If Factor X does not function properly, the probability of developing a chronic inflammatory disease increases.

At the same time, it is known that psychological stress can stimulate the inflammatory pathway that is inhibited by Factor X. For example, this can happen

19

through a stress-related leakiness of the intestinal wall, so that more bacteria from the intestine can penetrate into the bloodstream and into the lymph nodes in the abdominal cavity. Increased entry of bacteria into the abdominal cavity has been observed in psychological stress. These bacteria activate the Factor X pathway. So if there is now a disturbed function of Factor X and at the same time psychological stress is present, the inflammation intensifies. ◘ Figure 19.1 summarizes this fact again.

This convergence of two actually separate conditions, stress plus modified Factor X, has also been called the "double hit theory" of stress-related inflammation increase. There are further good indications for double hits when chronic inflammatory diseases and stress coincide.

We know very well that chronic inflammation means a relative increase in the activity of the sympathetic nervous system (▶ Chap. 17 "Sympathetic fires and causes high blood pressure"), while the cortisol stress axis functions largely normally. Since both stress axes work together—we called it cooperation of the stress axes—and both normally inhibit the immune system, the disturbance of this bilateral cooperation is a pro-inflammatory factor.

If stress now activates the stress axes, but the cooperation is disturbed, this can result in pro-inflammatory reactions. Conversely, chronic psychological stress can also disturb the cooperation of the stress axes, which can irritate some functions within the body (e.g. joint blood pressure regulation, joint blood sugar regulation, joint regulation of bronchial width in the lungs). ◘ Figure 19.2 summarizes the double hits.

After these explanations, it is now clear that psychological stress can exacerbate inflammation and that inflammation can also in turn impair brain performance, which is then experienced as stressful.

19.2 Anti-Stress Therapies

The last 10 years have brought new therapies from the field of psychology into the treatment of chronic inflammatory diseases. These include
- cognitive behavioral therapy,
- mindfulness and
- self-management.

All of them aim to ultimately better understand oneself and one's environment and then be able to react more appropriately. If stressful life circumstances can activate a chronic inflammatory disease, it is certainly very good if one can recognize the stress-triggering events early on in order to better adjust to them or even avoid them.

The author is not an expert in this field of psychology, but he recognizes that conventional medicine can learn a lot from psychologists. American universities and clinics are 10–15 years ahead of us in this respect. In Europe, the Dutch in particular started early with such psychological approaches. There are initial successes with these therapies for chronic inflammatory diseases. The number of studies on this topic has increased significantly.

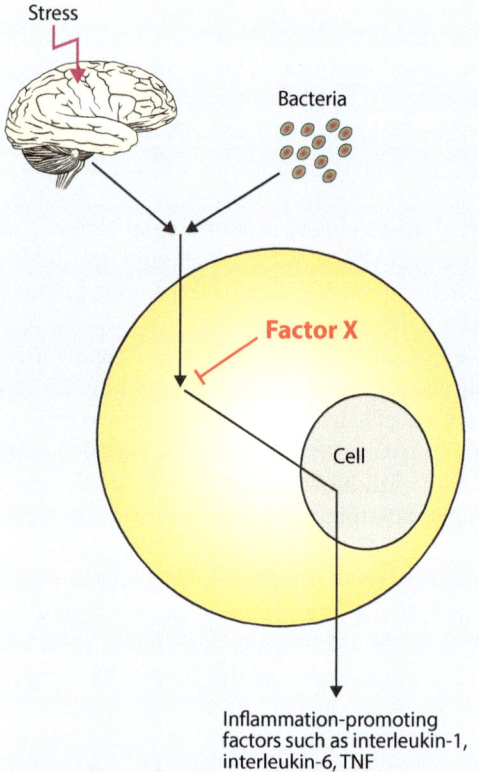

Importance of factor X in stress and inflammation. Bacteria stimulate an important cellular inflammatory pathway that contributes to the production of immune messengers such as interleukin-1, interleukin-6 and TNF. The same pathway can also be stimulated by psychological stress and also leads to an increase in immune messengers. Factor X inhibits this inflammatory pathway when it is working properly. If there is a genetic change in factor X, as can be the case with some chronic inflammatory diseases, the inflammatory pathway is no longer inhibited properly. Too many immune messengers are produced. So if a chronic inflammatory disease, a disturbed factor X and psychological stress come together, the inflammatory situation is intensified. This is also known as a "double hit."

■ **Fig. 19.1**   Significance of Factor X in stress and inflammation

19.3   Stress in the Elderly

19

In healthy people, stressful events are often associated with an increase in immune messengers in the blood. Interleukin-1 and Interleukin-6 are typically mentioned again and again. This fact has been studied even better in normal people than in

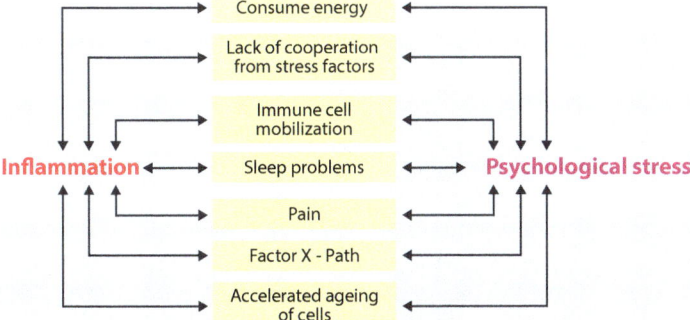

Double hit of mutual reinforcement of inflammation and psychological stress.

• Inflammation can consume energy and thus drain it from the brain during stress, which reduces brain
  performance (risk of chronic fatigue and depression, chap. 9). Conversely, stress can consume energy and
  disrupt a normal immune response.
• A lack of cooperation between the stress axes was discussed in the text.
• Inflammation can mobilize immune cells, and activated immune cells can disrupt the function
  of the brain and endocrine glands. Psychological stress can also mobilize immune
  cells, which can increase inflammation.
• Inflammation and psychological stress can cause sleep problems and thus exacerbate the energy
  shortage. Sleep problems also lead to inflammation and psychological stress.
• Inflammation stimulates pain and psychological stress exacerbates pain. Pain in turn increases
  inflammation and causes stress.
• The Factor X pathway was discussed in detail in the text and Fig. 19.1.
• Inflammation and stress cause premature ageing of various cells. Premature ageing, in turn, can be
  associated with disorders of immune cells and the brain.

Fig. 19.2 Double hit of mutual reinforcement of inflammation and psychological stress

patients with chronic inflammatory diseases. Therefore, the points mentioned in ▪ Fig. 19.2 are all applicable to normal people and normal aging. One point from ▪ Fig. 19.2, namely cell migration, will be discussed in more detail here.

Firdaus Dhabhar, a colleague from Miami University, once said that one should imagine the migration of immune cells as follows: "Redistribution of immune cells that come from the barracks, get onto the main roads and finally fight for the good on the battlefields."

Such mobilization or redistribution has undoubtedly been proven. There is a nice experiment with people who are parachuting for the first time in their life. It was conducted by Manfred Schedlowski (University of Duisburg-Essen) as early as the beginning of the 1990s.

It was found that special types of immune cells are released that are associated with the acute fight against infectious invaders. The stress-related migration of immune cells is therefore seen as a preparatory reaction to injury and risk of infection. Because migration of immune cells also means better surveillance of the body, as the mobilized immune cells can penetrate many tissues. And if more immune cells are on the move, penetrate various tissues, recognize infectious pathogens and release immune messengers in response (think for example of the intestinal wall and bacteria that have penetrated there), then the increased inflammatory situation can be explained, because the confrontation of the immune cells with, for example, bacteria triggers an inflammation.

Therefore, it is also true that many acute forms of stress in old age can be associated with an increase in inflammation. The example of an elderly person being relocated from their home environment to a nursing home was mentioned. There, the blood level of Interleukin-6 increased from the usual 2.5 pg/ml to 3.5 pg/ml (◨ Fig. 4.2). Even though many studies particularly examined the effects of acute stress on the increase in inflammation, it is also clear that chronic stress promotes inflammation. Here, the *caregiver stress* in the family care of a dementia patient is mentioned again. The *caregivers* suffer from chronic stress and higher inflammation, thus significantly increasing the risk of cardiovascular disease. Since these various reasons from ◨ Fig. 19.2 often occur together in the elderly, mutual reinforcement effects are likely.

The arrows in ◨ Fig. 19.2 show from stress to inflammation, but also vice versa, as inflammation also influences stress processing. In general, inflammation worsens stress processing or is even perceived as stress itself. In addition, inflammation can influence brain function in such a way that the onset of depression and dementia is accelerated or existing brain diseases are exacerbated. These relationships are well researched.

References

Bierhaus A, Wolf J, Andrassy M, Rohleder N, Humpert PM, Petrov D, Ferstl R, von EM, Wendt T, Rudofsky G, Joswig M, Morcos M, Schwaninger M, McEwen B, Kirschbaum C, Nawroth PP (2003) A mechanism converting psychosocial stress into mononuclear cell activation. Proc Natl Acad Sci U S A 100:1920–1925

Ghadban T, Schmidt-Yang M, Uzunoglu FG, Perez DR, El Gammal AT, Miro JT, Wellner U, Pantel K, Izbicki JR, Vashist YK (2015) Evaluation of the germline single nucleotide polymorphism rs583522 in the TNFAIP3 gene as a prognostic marker in esophageal cancer. Cancer Genet 208:595–601

Hassett AL, Epel E, Clauw DJ, Harris RE, Harte SE, Kairys A, Buyske S, Williams DA (2012) Pain is associated with short leukocyte telomere length in women with fibromyalgia. J Pain 13:959–969

Herrmann M, Schölmerich J, Straub RH (2000) Stress and rheumatic diseases. Rheum Dis Clin North Am 26:737–763

Kraaimaat FW, Brons MR, Geenen R, Bijlsma JW (1995) The effect of cognitive behavior therapy in patients with rheumatoid arthritis. Behav Res Ther 33:487–495

O'Donovan A, Tomiyama AJ, Lin J, Puterman E, Adler NE, Kemeny M, Wolkowitz OM, Blackburn EH, Epel ES (2012) Stress appraisals and cellular aging: a key role for anticipatory threat in the relationship between psychological stress and telomere length. Brain Behav Immun 26:573–579

Savolainen K, Eriksson JG, Kajantie E, Lahti M, Raikkonen K (2014) The history of sleep apnea is associated with shorter leukocyte telomere length: the Helsinki Birth Cohort Study. Sleep Med 15:209–212

Schedlowski M, Jacobs R, Alker J, Prohl F, Stratmann G, Richter S, Hadicke A, Wagner TO, Schmidt RE, Tewes U (1993) Psychophysiological, neuroendocrine and cellular immune reactions under psychological stress. Neuropsychobiology 28:87–90

Slavich GM, Irwin MR (2014) From stress to inflammation and major depressive disorder: a social signal transduction theory of depression. Psychol Bull 140: 774–815

Steptoe A, Hamer M, Chida Y (2007) The effects of acute psychological stress on circulating inflammatory factors in humans: a review and meta-analysis. Brain Behav Immun 21:901–912

Straub RH (2014) Rheumatoid arthritis: Stress in RA: a trigger of proinflammatory pathways? Nat Rev Rheumatol 10:516–518

Sturgeon JA, Finan PH, Zautra AJ (2016) Affective disturbance in rheumatoid arthritis: psychological and disease-related pathways. Nat Rev Rheumatol 10

Tempaku PF, Mazzotti DR, Tufik S (2015) Telomere length as a marker of sleep loss and sleep disturbances: a potential link between sleep and cellular senescence. Sleep Med 16:559–563

Zautra AJ, Davis MC, Reich JW, Nicassario P, Tennen H, Finan P, Kratz A, Parrish B, Irwin MR (2008) Comparison of cognitive behavioral and mindfulness meditation interventions on adaptation to rheumatoid arthritis for patients with and without history of recurrent depression. J Consult Clin Psychol 76:408–421

The Big Summary

The Synthesis

Contents

20.1   Addition of Energy Forms and Unwanted Energy
Expenditure – 196

20.2   What are Telomeres? – 198

20.3   Inflammation, Cell Turnover and Telomere
Length – 199

20.4   Chronic Inflammation and Telomere Length – 199

20.5   Pain, Stress and Telomere Length – 200

20.6   Anxiety, Smoking, and Telomere Length – 201

20.7   Conclusion – 202

References – 202

© The Author(s), under exclusive license to Springer-Verlag GmbH, DE, part of Springer Nature 2024
R. H. Straub, *Understanding Aging, Fatigue, and Inflammation*,
https://doi.org/10.1007/978-3-662-68904-2_20

20.1 Addition of Energy Forms and Unwanted Energy Expenditure

So far, energy expenditures have been presented in an integrated sense as follows:

We consume a certain amount of energy with food and expend it for various activities, with the main part being used for the basal metabolic rate including heat production and food processing, and this is about 60–85% depending on age. The remaining energy is used for voluntarily desired energy expenditures in the form of physical or mental activity. These figures are average values of the normal population, as used in ◘ Fig. 8.2 in ▶ Chap. 8 ("What does increased energy expenditure mean for the body?"). The individual energy expenditures add up in an additive sense, so one could also write:

Total expenditure = Basal metabolic rate + Food processing + Desired physical/mental activity

This makes the energy considerations relatively simple, because it is essentially about the mathematical addition or subtraction of energy forms that determine the final result—the total energy expenditure. However, if an additional unwanted energy expenditure is added to the above equation, then the formula looks like this:

Total expenditure = Basal metabolic rate + Food processing
+ Desired physical/mental activity
+ **unwanted energy expenditure**

In this equation, the total expenditure and the basal metabolic rate remain approximately the same and the energy expenditure caused by food intake (for digestion) only slightly decreases (due to loss of appetite), the desired energy expenditure for physical/mental actions is reduced by the unwanted energy expenditures. Herman Pontzer recognized an upper limit of total energy expenditure that is far away from the intestinal absorptive capacity of 20000 kJ/day. He called it "constraint total energy expenditure". With this constraint, the individual reaches a level of energy expenditure above which he usually does not spend more energy. The constraint situation explains why every unwanted energy expenditure must reduce energy expenditure for the desired things.

In the case of chronic inflammatory disease, this reduction is crucially determined by the activated immune system, with elements such as disease-related stress, pain, sleep problems, and so on playing an additional role. This relationship was clearly demonstrated in rheumatoid arthritis. During aging, other unwanted energy expenditures such as chronic pain, chronic psychological stress, excessive smoking, sleep problems, anxiety/fear, and chronic smoldering infections are considered.

The consequences are similar in chronic inflammatory diseases and during aging, as there is a reduction in the desired physical/mental activity. This reduction in physical/mental activity is associated with complications that manifest as daytime fatigue, sleep disorders, loss of appetite, muscle loss and obesity, bone loss, insulin resistance, declining libido, high blood pressure, increased blood clotting, cardiovascular diseases, age-related diabetes, depression, dementia, decreased immune surveillance and therefore also cancer.

Regarding the last point, the following should be added: It is clear today that the immune system is essential in the recognition of cancer cells. Cancer cells have foreign proteins on their surface that are recognized as foreign by cells of the immune system. This leads to a local defense reaction of the immune cells, and the cancer cells are killed. If the immune system does not function properly or if immune surveillance is poor, the development of cancer can be promoted.

Usually, these complications are attributed to aging problems because they rarely affect young people (however, they do in chronic inflammatory diseases in childhood or early to middle adulthood). However, they do not necessarily have to be present in the elderly, and it is the goal of geriatric research and care to influence this. Elderly people should live as long as possible in good health, so that the phase of illness and subsequent death is as short as possible. This is often represented as in ◘ Fig. 20.1.

The presentation in this book could be called integrated or holistic, as it largely left individual details of the molecular relationships unmentioned. Holistic had a negative connotation a few decades ago because such an approach was considered unscientific and "un-molecular". However, energy considerations, evolutionary medicine, hormonal and neuronal networks (brain!) and cytokine networks (immune system!) provide a scientific platform that can answer ultimate questions in a holistic sense (see preface).

The text should remain readable, and this is achieved with a superordinate approach, so that the key points can be understood by everyone. However, this superordinate approach must not be unscientific. With this, the book could actually end. But to give a last molecular insight in this book, let's point out the connection between energy and aging from a completely different perspective.

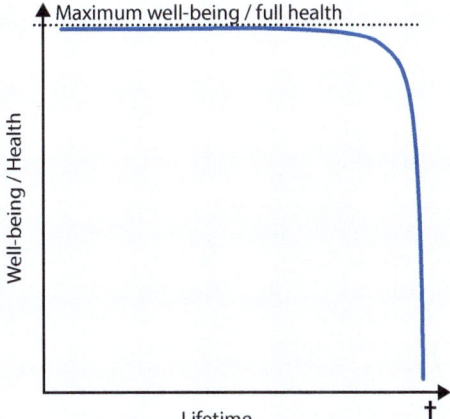

Optimal relationship between lifespan and well-being/health. It is optimal to be very healthy for as long as possible. Only shortly before death (†) does the phase of health end suddenly, and there is a rapid end without prolonged infirmity.

◘ **Fig. 20.1**   Optimal relationship between lifetime and well-being/health

20.2 What are Telomeres?

Elisabeth Blackburn is an Australian molecular biologist who grew up in the remote Tasmania, then studied in Melbourne and Cambridge, went to the USA to conduct science in the major universities of this country (Yale, Berkeley, Stanford, San Diego-La Jolla). In 1984, she worked with her then doctoral student Carol Greider on an important element at the long end of the chromosome, the telomere (Greek *telos*, the end; Greek meros, the part).

The telomeres consist of repeating units of the genetic substance DNA (◘ Fig. 20.2). When these repeating pieces become increasingly smaller over the course of cell life, this indicates cell aging. Since pretty much all cells in all living beings age, the shortening telomeres are a widely accepted phenomenon of cell aging. The shortening of telomere length and cell aging are thus a completely normal thing during aging.

The shortening of the telomeres at the end of the chromosomes has an opponent named telomerase (◘ Fig. 20.2). The enzyme telomerase was also described by Elisabeth Blackburn and Carol Greider, and they were honored with the Nobel

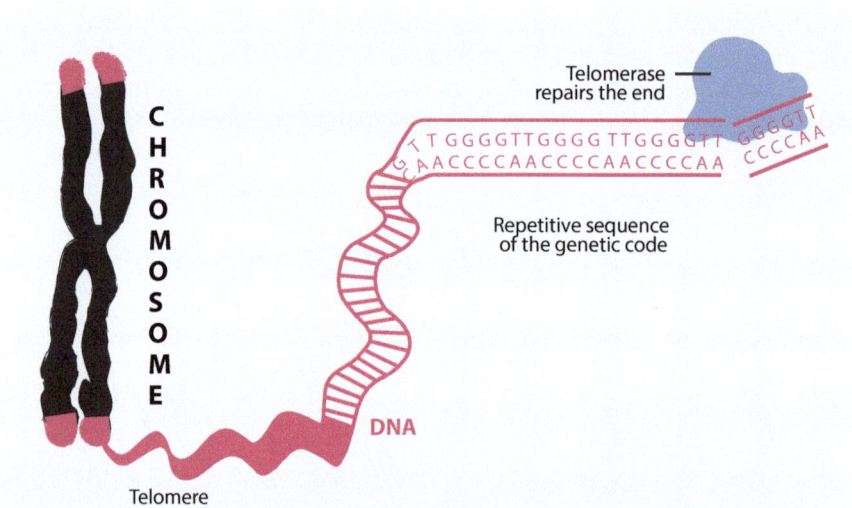

Telomere and telomerase. On the left, the chromosome is shown in black, with the pink caps of the telomere at its ends. The diagram shows how the DNA (genetic material) is composed in the area of the telomere (the pink-colored area). The resolution increases steadily from left to right until the individual letters (A, C, G, T) of the genetic code can be recognized on the right. The double-stranded DNA is enlarged from left to right and the details become more and more visible. The telomere is always made up of the same DNA sections, so that the sequence of the genetic code in the telomere is constantly repeated. The blue telomerase is shown on the right, which extends the end of the telomere so that the overall length of the telomere remains as constant as possible. The telomerase attaches pieces of DNA that correspond exactly to the repeating code of the telomere.

◘ **Fig. 20.2**   Telomere and Telomerase

Prize for this work on the telomere in 2009. The enzyme telomerase ensures the extension of the telomeres and thus works against the cellular aging process.

Furthermore, this anti-aging enzyme stabilizes the function of the mitochondria, the power plants of the cell, which we got to know in ▶ Chap. 1 "Energy and Body". With this mitochondria-protecting function, telomerase is important for cellular energy supply and cell survival. In addition, telomerase supports the production of the universal energy coin ATP in the mitochondrion, so it is directly involved in energy production. If telomerase does not function properly, premature aging can occur, and the telomeres are then significantly shortened. If telomerase is artificially introduced into an otherwise telomerase-poor cell, the lifespan of this cell can be significantly increased.

With these preliminary considerations, we now ask ourselves whether the unwanted energy expenditures described in Part II "Energy Expenditures in the Spotlight" have anything to do with telomere length or cell aging.

20.3 Inflammation, Cell Turnover and Telomere Length

Inflammations always lead to a higher turnover of immune cells. This mechanism was preserved (positively selected) in the evolutionary process to generate a suitable cellular immune response in infectious diseases. We had already learned about this adaptation process in ▶ Chap. 3 under "Energy Storage—Long-term Roles of Brain and Immune System" in the context of vaccination. In vaccinations, the immune response to the pathogen (foreign antigen) should also fit as perfectly as possible, and for this a high cell turnover is needed. A high cell turnover guarantees the highest possible adaptation to the foreign antigen.

In this respect, an aging process of the immune cells, which is expected with high cell turnover, is desired, so that the less well-adapted immune cells die quickly and make room for the better adapted immune cells. During an infection process, the number of matching immune cells typically increases until day 14. Now the infection can be overcome, and afterwards the immune cells die off again until day 21. The entire process is accompanied by significant shortening of the telomeres as a sign of high turnover and immune cell aging. Inflammation is thus closely associated with shortened telomeres.

But what happens when the inflammation is of a chronic nature?

20.4 Chronic Inflammation and Telomere Length

In the animal model of chronic malaria infection in a native songbird—the siskin (*Spinus*)—the length of the telomeres in the cells of various tissues is significantly shortened. This suggests accelerated cell aging in the chronic inflammation caused by malaria. In chronic liver inflammation caused by the hepatitis virus, a significant shortening of the telomeres is also observed, leading to premature aging of immune cells.

In chronic inflammatory diseases in humans, the telomeres in the immune cells are often shortened. A reduction in telomerase activity plays an important role in this. Chronic inflammatory diseases are often accompanied by inflammatory flare-ups with varying lengths of free intervals. Here, one can then imagine a rise and fall of immune cell aging.

In summary, it can be said that the unwanted energy expenditure of acute and chronic inflammation is associated with a shortening of telomeres in white blood cells, aging of immune cells, but also with aging of the tissues affected by the inflammation.

20.5 Pain, Stress and Telomere Length

The relationship between pain and increased inflammation has already been demonstrated. The pain nerve fibers themselves are capable of triggering a local inflammation when activated in a certain area—for example, in the skin. Remember your last bee sting! When the bee sinks its stinger into the skin, it releases toxins there. These toxins spread in the skin tissue and encounter the nerve ending of a pain fiber, as shown in ◘ Fig. 5.1. Now the pain fiber is stimulated, and it sends a signal to the spinal cord and brain, so we consciously perceive the bee sting.

At the same time, the pain nerve fibers release neurotransmitters that increase inflammation and swelling (this was labeled as "NT" in the legend of ◘ Fig. 5.1). So, pain is often associated with an increased inflammatory situation, and conversely, local inflammation also causes pain. In addition, pain has also been linked to shortened telomere length. Patients with a chronic pain condition (fibromyalgia) have shortened telomeres. If depression is also present, the shortening of the telomeres is particularly pronounced. Chronic pain combined with the normal age-related telomere shortening thus represents a "double hit". Together with depression, it is a "triple hit."

When people now experience psychological stress and perceive it as threatening, as can happen, for example, when caring for Alzheimer's patients, the telomere length in the examined white blood cells of these caring family members is shortened. According to all that has been said so far, this means accelerated cell aging of the white blood cells in psychological stress. Such cell aging is then probably associated with higher inflammation, because increased aging also means increased cleanup of dead white blood cells. Such cleanup actions can show up as an increased inflammatory situation in the blood. In this way, the already existing cellular aging process and additional psychological stress could mutually reinforce each other. This principle can also be referred to as a "double hit."

Even with the psychological stress of shift work, the telomere lengths in white blood cells are shortened. A study also showed that a long sleep duration was associated with longer telomeres. The situation is very similar with other types in sleep disorders, as these have also been linked to shortened telomere length in white blood cells. The increase in sleep problems is evident in phases with sleep apnea. This sleep apnea is associated with shortened telomeres in white blood cells.

Even if these phenomena in white blood cells do not speak for the whole body, and even if these phenomena in the white blood cells may not have been studied over a longer period of time, there is at least some evidence for the connection between telomere length and sleep problems. This situation can also be a "double hit", where natural aging and simultaneous sleep problems can lead to an increase in the cellular aging process.

20.6 Anxiety, Smoking, and Telomere Length

A study from Groningen in the Netherlands showed the correlation between anxiety and the shortening of telomeres in white blood cells. Over 900 people were examined twice over a period of 2 years. At the beginning of the study, anxiety was assessed using a questionnaire, and two years later, the telomere lengths in the white blood cells were measured. Those individuals with a high degree of anxiety had shorter telomeres. The correlation between anxiety and shortened telomeres has been demonstrated several times. Since anxious people also sleep worse and experience a higher degree of stress, the shortening of telomeres could be triggered by "multiple hits".

In a more recent Dutch study, a correlation was found between smoking and short telomeres in white blood cells. This indicates premature aging of immune cells triggered by smoking. This study confirms previous studies on smokers, where a clear relationship was found between the number of cigarettes per day and telomere shortening in white blood cells. An English study showed the correlation between the number of smoking years and telomere shortening, with long-term smoking associated with greater shortening or cell aging.

We can summarize at this point that the unwanted energy expenditures described in Part II "Energy Expenditures in the Spotlight" have a direct influence on telomere length. These unwanted energy expenditures are shown in ◘ Table 20.1.

One could also phrase it differently, that unwanted energy expenditures accelerate the aging of white blood cells—i.e., immune cells. At this point, we do not know exactly whether this also applies to other cells of the body. However, some findings suggest that with one or another unwanted energy expenditure, other cells such as

◘ **Table 20.1**   Unwanted energy expenditures as a percentage of total energy expenditure

Situation[*]	Additional energy expenditure
Acute pain (electric shocks to the abdominal skin)	up to 65% more
Chronic pain	up to 15% more
Psychological stress	up to 30% more
Anxiety/Fear	up to 10% more
Sleep disorders	up to 30% more
Chronic smoldering infections	up to 10% more
Chronic smoking (more than 6 cigarettes/day)	up to 15% more

[*] The individual situations should not be considered independently of each other, as pain can be linked with sleep disorders or anxiety with psychological stress, etc. Therefore, the percentages cannot simply be added together to calculate the total increase in additional energy expenditure

vascular wall cells or heart muscle cells also age faster. The example of chronic malaria in the siskin (*Spinus*) demonstrates this in animal experiments.

We now recognize that unwanted energy expenditures shorten telomeres, which is caused by the reduction in the activity of the anti-aging enzyme telomerase. We have learned that telomerase is closely linked to the functioning of cellular energy production. With these preliminary considerations, one can now summarize this book in a few sentences.

20.7 Conclusion

Unwanted energy expenditures divert energy from the entire system, which is not available for desired energy expenditures such as physical and mental activity (holistically). At the same time, unwanted energy expenditures reduce the activity of the anti-aging enzyme telomerase, leading to cell aging and cellular energy shortages (molecularly). Since the mentioned systems are closely intertwined, one should not assume a single triggering factor when exacerbating energy shortages. On the contrary, the logic of "double hits" and "multiple hits" tells us that several unwanted factors contribute to the overall problem simultaneously or successively and may possibly reinforce each other.

The view on energy balance and evolutionary medicine made it clear that all double and multiple hits for short-term energy-consuming reactions were preserved during evolution. In this process, the two egoists—the brain and the immune system—constantly fight over energy reserves. However, they also cooperate in the short term (mutual immediate assistance). They dominate the energy consumption of unwanted and desired energy expenditures. They use very different mechanisms. The brain essentially uses hormones and nerve pathways, especially the stress axes, the immune system uses immune messengers (= cytokines) and circulating immune cells.

The long-term or chronic use of the actually short-term intended programs unfortunately leads to unwanted energy shortages, reduced physical/mental activity, accelerated aging, and chronic resultant problems.

So, if we want to properly treat patients with long-lasting inflammatory diseases, we need to consider and possibly treat the various unwanted energy expenditures. It is not enough to just block the inflammation. In chronic inflammatory diseases and during aging, the various possibilities of unwanted energy expenditures must be minimized in order to maintain physical and mental activity at a high level.

References

Ale-Agha N, Dyballa-Rukes N, Jakob S, Altschmied J, Haendeler J (2014) Cellular functions of the dual-targeted catalytic subunit of telomerase, telomerase reverse transcriptase—potential role in senescence and aging. Exp Gerontol 56:189–193

Asghar M, Palinauskas V, Zaghdoudi-Allan N, Valkiunas G, Mukhin A, Platonova E, Farnert A, Bensch S, Hasselquist D (2016) Parallel telomere shortening in multiple body tissues owing to malaria infection. Proc Biol Sci 283:20161184

Barcelo A, Pierola J, Lopez-Escribano H, de la Pena M, Soriano JB, Alonso-Fernandez A, Ladaria A, Agusti A (2010) Telomere shortening in sleep apnea syndrome. Respir Med 104:1225–1229

Damjanovic AK, Yang Y, Glaser R, Kiecolt-Glaser JK, Nguyen H, Laskowski B, Zou Y, Beversdorf DQ, Weng NP (2007) Accelerated telomere erosion is associated with a declining immune function of caregivers of Alzheimer's disease patients. J Immunol 179:4249–4254

Georgin-Lavialle S, Aouba A, Mouthon L, Londono-Vallejo JA, Lepelletier Y, Gabet AS, Hermine O (2010) The telomere/telomerase system in autoimmune and systemic immune-mediated diseases. Autoimmun Rev 9:646–651

Hassett AL, Epel E, Clauw DJ, Harris RE, Harte SE, Kairys A, Buyske S, Williams DA (2012) Pain is associated with short leukocyte telomere length in women with fibromyalgia. J Pain 13:959–969

Hoen PW, Rosmalen JG, Schoevers RA, Huzen J, van der Harst P, de JP (2013) Association between anxiety but not depressive disorders and leukocyte telomere length after 2 years of follow-up in a population-based sample. Psychol Med 43:689–697

Huzen J, Wong LS, van Veldhuisen DJ, Samani NJ, Zwinderman AH, Codd V, Cawthon RM, Benus GF, van der Horst IC, Navis G, Bakker SJ, Gansevoort RT, de Jong PE, Hillege HL, van Gilst WH, de Boer RA, van der Harst P (2014) Telomere length loss due to smoking and metabolic traits. J Intern Med 275:155–163

Liang G, Schernhammer E, Qi L, Gao X, De V, I, Han J (2011) Associations between rotating night shifts, sleep duration, and telomere length in women. PLoS One 6:e23462

Munsterman T, Takken T, Wittink H (2012) Are persons with rheumatoid arthritis deconditioned? A review of physical activity and aerobic capacity. BMC Musculoskelet Disord 13:202–213

Najarro K, Nguyen H, Chen G, Xu M, Alcorta S, Yao X, Zukley L, Metter EJ, Truong T, Lin Y, Li H, Oelke M, Xu X, Ling SM, Longo DL, Schneck J, Leng S, Ferrucci L, Weng NP (2015) Telomere Length as an Indicator of the Robustness of B- and T-Cell Response to Influenza in Older Adults. J Infect Dis 212:1261–1269

Okereke OI, Prescott J, Wong JY, Han J, Rexrode KM, De VI, (2012) High phobic anxiety is related to lower leukocyte telomere length in women. PLoS One 7:e40516

Pontzer H (2018). Energy Constraint as a Novel Mechanism Linking Exercise and Health. Physiology (Bethesda). 33:384–393

Rudolph KL, Chang S, Lee HW, Blasco M, Gottlieb GJ, Greider C, DePinho RA (1999) Longevity, stress response, and cancer in aging telomerase-deficient mice. Cell 96:701–712

Straub RH (2017). The brain and immune system prompt energy shortage in chronic inflammation and ageing. Nat Rev Rheumatol. 13:743–751

Tempaku PF, Mazzotti DR, Tufik S (2015) Telomere length as a marker of sleep loss and sleep disturbances: a potential link between sleep and cellular senescence. Sleep Med 16:559–563

Valdes AM, Andrew T, Gardner JP, Kimura M, Oelsner E, Cherkas LF, Aviv A, Spector TD (2005) Obesity, cigarette smoking, and telomere length in women. Lancet 366:662–664

Supplementary Information

Appendix – 206

Appendix

▪ Glossary

Abscess - A collection of white blood cells and bacteria (*pus*) in a cavity that has formed by the melting of previously healthy tissue. Abscesses can primarily occur in the skin, but also at all other locations. They are hardly treatable with antibiotic therapy. They must be surgically opened and drained.

Adrenal gland, cortex and medulla - The adrenal glands are glands that sit like little caps on the kidneys. They each have the size of an apricot, and they produce various hormones that are released into the bloodstream. The adrenal cortex is distinguished, from which cortisol and androgens originate. In the adrenal cortex, an important hormone for blood pressure regulation is also produced. In addition, the adrenal medulla is distinguished, which is surrounded by the cortex (similar to the apricot kernel by the apricot flesh). Adrenaline is produced in the adrenal medulla. Adrenaline is the number 1 stress hormone. The brain is the supreme master of the adrenal gland, which hormonally activates the adrenal cortex via the pituitary gland and the adrenal medulla via the sympathetic nervous system. The adrenal cortex and adrenal medulla belong to the stress system.

Allele - The allele from the direct male ancestor (father) and the allele from the direct female ancestor (mother) are alternative forms of the same gene. The dominant allele, in contrast to the recessive allele, leads to trait formation.

Andropause - The andropause describes the male menopause (gr. andrós, man). It occurs somewhat later than the menopause of women (around the 50th year of life). The andropause is associated with an increasingly lower production of male sex hormones. Although men generally retain the ability to procreate into old age, the probability significantly decreases of still producing enough fertile sperm to father offspring.

Antibody - Antibodies are produced by immune cells (more specifically by plasma cells). Antibodies always target antigens. In many cases, this leads to the neutralization of the antigen and the uptake and destruction of the antigen by phagocytes.

Antigens - Antigens are recognized and attacked by our immune system as foreign. Antigens are often structures located on the surface of bacteria or viruses (e.g., tetanus toxin). The attack is carried out with precisely matching antibodies and immune cells with precisely matching surface structures (we have already referred to them as antennas of the immune cells). Autoantigens are referred to when the antigens consist of the body's own material (hence auto), against which a immune reaction and an inflammatory reaction are mistakenly initiated.

Arteriosclerosis - Arteriosclerosis is also called arterial calcification. It is a disease of the walls of the arteries (arteries) with increasing hardening (proliferation of connective tissue), inflammation, and deposition of blood fats and calcium. It is the platform for the formation of sudden blood clots, which can detach (embolism) or completely block the vessel (heart attack, stroke, vascular occlusion).

ATP - Adenosine triphosphate is the universally valid energy currency that is produced in the mitochondria. A molecule of ATP consists of 10 carbon atoms, 16 hydrogen atoms, 5 nitrogen atoms, 13 oxygen atoms, and precisely 3 (hence triphosphate) phosphorus atoms. ATP is needed for many cellular metabolic steps and for cell construction. The production of a single protein molecule of medium size requires approximately 2000 ATP molecules.

Basal metabolic rate: - It refers to the amount of energy required in absolute rest in a warm bed in the morning. It serves the basic supply of all organs and organ systems. The basal metabolic rate cannot be negotiated (see also CAEN).

CAEN - "Controllable amount of energy" or controllable quantity of energy. Under the conditions in the warm bed, the cells draw their basic needs from the flowing blood. Below a certain basal metabolic range, the organs do not negotiate among themselves. In a human body, much is indicated with the intestinal absorptive capacity, so 20,000 kJ (4777 kcal). Little is indicated with the basal metabolic rate, which is not negotiated, so about 7500 kJ (1791 kcal). The calculated difference between the intestinal absorptive capacity and the basal metabolic rate, which is roughly 20,000 kJ minus 7500 kJ = 12,500 kJ (2986 kcal), can be negotiated. We call it here the controllable amount of energy.

Castor and Pollux - Castor was the mortal son of Tyndareus, King of Sparta, and his wife Leda; Pollux was the immortal son of Zeus and Leda. Zeus seduced Leda in the form of a swan.

Chronic obstructive pulmonary disease - COPD (chronic obstructive pulmonary disease; obstructive = blocking) refers to a disease with increasing narrowing and mucus-related blockage of the bronchi. This can often occur after years of smoking, leading to smoker's lung. Other causes can be of an allergic nature, as in allergic asthma. The increasing blockage leads to lung overinflation and structural remodeling of the lung in the form of scarring and a reduction in the gas exchange surface.

Cortisol - Cortisol is the active hormone of the adrenal cortex. It is not cortisone, which is often substituted for it in common parlance. Cortisol is a stress hormone of the selfish brain. It leads to the release of energy-rich substrates from stores such as adipose tissue and the liver. Thus, cortisol can increase the levels of fatty acids and sugar in the blood. At the same time, it has anti-inflammatory effects.

Cytokines - Cytokines are the messenger substances of immune cells and other cells that are intended to act in the immediate vicinity of the cells. We could also call cytokines messenger substances for the immediate neighborhood or neighbor's messenger substance (see also messenger substances). Some cytokines have long-range effects (e.g., interleukin-6).

Diabetes mellitus - Diabetes, i.e., the sugar levels in the blood are too high. In type 1 diabetes mellitus, there is an autoimmune disease in which the immune system recognizes proteins of the insulin-producing pancreas as "foreign". Due to the inflammation-related demise of insulin production, these patients need insulin as a permanent therapy. These patients are usually younger. In type 2 diabetes mellitus (age-related diabetes), on the other hand, insulin production remains intact for a long time until it dries up after years of overproduction (exhaustion of the pancreas). The latter disease is not an autoimmune disease.

Emaciation time - The time that would pass until death due to, for example, an infection, if we were to live only from our energy stores. In the case of infections, a small amount of energy can be absorbed in the form of fluids, but the usual energy intake is significantly restricted.

Epidemiology - Epidemiology is the "science of the origin, spread, control, and social consequences of epidemics, typical mass diseases of the time, and damages of civilization."

Factor X - Here, the factor is simply called "Factor X" so that one does not have to remember the complicated name "TNF alpha induced protein 3" (TNFAIP3). Anyone who wants to know more can find Factor X under this name on the internet.

Glucose - Glucose, or dextrose, is an important basic unit of carbohydrates. Glucose is a crucial energy-rich substrate, particularly used for ATP (energy) production under low-oxygen conditions. Glucose can be stored in the form of starch in the liver, kidneys, and muscles.

Hyperinsulinemia - Hyperinsulinemia means high blood levels of the hormone insulin, which goes hand in hand with insulin resistance.

Immunomodulators - See Cytokines.

Insulin - It is the storage hormone par excellence originating from the pancreas, as it promotes the uptake of both glucose and fatty acids into the storage organs (adipose tissue, skeletal muscles, liver). Furthermore, it is a growth factor for many tissues, including the immune system. Diabetics with high blood glucose levels receive therapeutic insulin to lower the glucose in the blood and transport it into the storage organs.

Interleukin - For example, Interleukin-1 or Interleukin-6. These are cytokines that are intended to act in the immediately adjacent area (local effect). Some cytokines like Interleukin-6 also have distant effects, as they can be transported to far distant locations via the circulation in the vessels (see Cytokines).

Ion pump - Ions are, for example, sodium or calcium, which are excreted in the kidney. The pumping out or pumping in of ions from/into cells is costly. Pumping costs about 10–25% of the energy made available in the cell. Such pumps are switched on

when sweating, which is why more energy is expended at high temperatures.

Jason and the Argonauts - Jason and the Argonauts sought the Golden Fleece. In mythology, it is the skin of a golden ram that could fly and speak. From today's perspective, according to one theory, these were sheepskins that were used for gold panning in the gold-rich Colchis in the western Caucasus.

Macular Degeneration - Macular degeneration refers to the destruction of an important section of the retina, referred to as the "point of sharpest vision", namely the macula. This leads to a decrease in central visual acuity with increasingly severe visual impairment.

Messenger substances - Messenger substances mediate between distant organs, but also between closely adjacent cells. Between the organs, the nerve fibers and their neurotransmitters are relevant, such as noradrenaline (in the ending of the sympathetic nerve fiber). Hormones also mediate between organs, for example between the pituitary gland and the adrenal glands, which then produce cortisol. Between closely adjacent cells, the cytokines (from ancient Greek kýtos jar; kinos movement) mediate, which are produced for the purpose of local cell communication. Sometimes, however, such cytokines can also mediate between organs, which is the case, for example, for interleukin-6.

Mitochondria - Mitochondria are the energy producers of our cells. They produce ATP (Adenosine triphosphate), which is the energy currency that can be used virtually everywhere, which is why ATP production is constantly and universally ongoing.

Mutation - The genetic material, despite its high constancy, is subject to individual, spontaneously arisen genetic changes. Permanent genetic changes are called mutations. A mutation can lead to a new trait or a modification of a trait. Example: One or more mutations are responsible for moths suddenly having dark gray wings instead of white wings.

Noradrenaline - Noradrenaline is primarily a neurotransmitter of the sympathetic nerve fiber. When noradrenaline is considered in flowing blood, it is sometimes called a hormone. In addition, immune cells can produce noradrenaline locally, so it could also be referred to as a cytokine (it has not been referred to as a cytokine so far) (see also sympathetic nervous system).

Obesity - Obesity = excessive fatness is defined as a Body Mass Index of equal or more than 30 kg/m^2 (Body Mass Index = weight in kg divided by height in m squared). People are called normal weight if the Body Mass Index is between 18.5 and 25 kg/m^2. Between 25 and 30 kg/m^2 it is called overweight.

Parasympathetic Nervous System - The counterpart of the sympathetic nervous system. Where the sympathetic nervous system is responsible for fight and flight, the parasympathetic nervous system is responsible for digestion and the absorption of energy-rich substrates (glucose, fats, amino acids). The parasympathetic and sympathetic nervous systems are opponents: when one system is more active, the other is quite inactive.

Proximate - One could translate "proximate" as "immediately nearby" and "ultimate" as "fundamental".

RAA Hormones - The RAA hormones **R**enin, **A**ngiotensin and **A**ldosterone have a primary role in increasing blood pressure. During stressful events, blood pressure needs to rise. The sympathetic nervous system, with its neurotransmitters noradrenaline and adrenaline, stimulates the RAA hormone system. The RAA hormone system and the sympathetic nervous system increase blood pressure by reducing the excretion of water in the kidney and constricting the vessels. The excess water thus remains in the constricted vessel system, which increases blood pressure.

Rheumatoid Arthritis - Inflammation of multiple joints, usually of the hands and feet, but also of the large joints and the spine. The disease can also affect tissues outside the joints. It is an autoimmune disease, in which the immune system mistakenly recognizes the body's own tissue as foreign and attacks it. Since the immune system is active, these patients need more energy for this immune system.

Selection, positively selected - The individuals better adapted to their respective environment have a greater probability of surviving in the competition. They are "selected" from the multitude of possibilities. We say of a species that still exists today that it has been positively selected or has experienced positive selection. This means that the species or a trait of this species (e.g., red comb in roosters) underwent positive selection after many generations, so the species or the trait is still there; it was positively selected. In contrast, all species that no longer exist today and have become extinct have undergone negative selection; they were negatively selected.

Shear forces - Shear forces are obliquely acting forces that can have a damaging effect on the vessel wall.

Sickness Behavior - *Sickness behavior*, for example in infectious disease (flu). *Sickness behavior* manifests itself in the form of discomfort, daytime fatigue, exhaustion, lack of drive, increased feeling of cold, muscle pain, joint pain, loss of appetite, anxiety, depressive feelings, retreat into familiar safe areas, and lack of energy.

Stress axes - The stress axes are activated during acute stress. They serve the acute redistribution of energy-rich substrates from the stores (fat tissue, muscles, liver) to the consumers (brain, muscles, heart muscle, immune system). Essentially, it is about the brain-pituitary-adrenal axis (end product: cortisol) and the brain-sympathetic nervous system axis (end products: adrenaline from the adrenal gland and noradrenaline from the sympathetic nerve fibers). In times of stress, the thyroid hormones and the RAA hormones (see there) are also released.

Symbiosis - Symbiosis is the coexistence of two living beings that is beneficial for both partners.

Sympathetic Nervous System - It is the central stress system of the human body with the two neurotransmitters adrenaline and noradrenaline. Adrenaline originates from the adrenal medulla. The nerve fibers of the sympathetic nervous system are called sympathetic nerve fibers, which are virtually present everywhere in the body (exception: placenta). Noradrenaline is located in the endings of the sympathetic nerve fibers.

TNF - TNF stands for Tumor Necrosis Factor, because this cytokine can destroy tumors. When it was first described, this tumor-destroying property was predominant. Today, TNF is considered one of the most important pro-inflammatory factors of the activated immune system. It is released when, for example, a bacterium reacts with a receptor on the surface of an immune cell.

Trier Social Stress Test (TSST) - A popular method of acutely inducing stress in humans is an unprepared speech in front of an "important" examination committee, where the performance can allegedly decide on professional advancement. The test is called the Trier Social Stress Test (TSST) because it was invented at the University of Trier, Germany. This test is used worldwide today.

Thymus - The thymus is an organ of the immune system located in the chest cavity below the breastbone and slightly above the heart, about the size of a peach. There, a specific type of immune cells is trained, which is called T-cell (T as in Thymus).

Ultimate - One could translate "ultimate" as "fundamental" and "proximate" as "immediately nearby".

Vagus nerve - The vagus nerve is the main nerve of the parasympathetic nervous system, controlling the digestive system. It originates in medulla oblongata within the skull, and it is significantly responsible for the continuous movement of the stomach and intestines. It also promotes the release of digestive enzymes and insulin from the pancreas. It supplies the intestine up to the middle of the large intestine. According to new research, the large intestine—especially concerning the release of stool—is mainly subject to the sympathetic nervous system.